Fluids and Electrolytes

Editor

JOSHUA SQUIERS

NURSING CLINICS
OF NORTH AMERICA

www.nursing.theclinics.com

Consulting Editor
STEPHEN D. KRAU

June 2017 • Volume 52 • Number 2

ELSEVIER

1600 John F. Kennedy Boulevard ● Suite 1800 ● Philadelphia, Pennsylvania, 19103-2899

http://www.theclinics.com

NURSING CLINICS OF NORTH AMERICA Volume 52, Number 2
June 2017 ISSN 0029-6465, ISBN-13: 978-0-323-50981-7

Editor: Kerry Holland
Developmental Editor: Casey Potter

Nursing Clinics of North America (ISSN 0029-6465) is published quarterly by Elsevier Inc., 360 Park Avenue South, New York, NY 10010-1710. Months of issue are March, June, September, and December. Periodicals postage paid at New York, NY and additional mailing offices. Subscription price per year is, $155.00 (US individuals), $465.00 (US institutions), $275.00 (international individuals), $567.00 (international institutions), $220.00 (Canadian individuals), $567.00 (Canadian institutions), $100.00 (US students), and $135.00 (international students). To receive student/resident rate, orders must be accompanied by name of affiliated institution, date of term, and the signature of program/residency coordinator on institution letterhead. Orders will be billed at individual rate until proof of status is received. Foreign air speed delivery is included in all *Clinics* subscription prices. All prices are subject to change without notice. **POSTMASTER:** Send address changes to *Nursing Clinics*, Elsevier Health Sciences Division, Subscription Customer Service, 3251 Riverport Lane, Maryland Heights, MO 63043. **Customer Service: Telephone: 1-800-654-2452** (U.S. and Canada); **1-314-447-8871 (outside U.S. and Canada). Fax: 1-314-447-8029. E-mail: journalscustomerservice-usa@elsevier.com** (for print support) and **journalsonlinesupport-usa@elsevier.com** (for online support).

Nursing Clinics of North America is covered in *EMBASE/Excerpta Medica, MEDLINE/PubMed (Index Medicus), Social Sciences Citation Index, Current Contents, ASCA, Cumulative Index to Nursing, RNdex Top 100,* and Allied Health Literature and International Nursing Index (INI).

Contributors

CONSULTING EDITOR

STEPHEN D. KRAU, PhD, RN, CNE
Associate Professor, School of Nursing, Vanderbilt University, Nashville, Tennessee

EDITOR

JOSHUA SQUIERS, PhD, ACNP-BC, AGACNP-BC, FCCM
Assistant Professor of Nursing, Oregon Health and Science University School of Nursing, Director of the Acute Care Nurse Practitioner Program (AGACNP), Assistant Professor of Anesthesiology, Oregon Health and Science University School of Medicine, Division of Cardiac and Surgical Subspecialty Critical Care, Department of Anesthesiology and Perioperative Medicine, Portland, Oregon

AUTHORS

NATHAN E. ASHBY, MD
Assistant Professor of Clinical Anesthesiology and Critical Care, Adjunct Assistant Professor of Nursing, Department of Anesthesiology, Division of Critical Care, Vanderbilt University Medical Center, Nashville, Tennessee

BROOKE A. BAILEY, DNP, AGACNP, CNS
Department of Advanced Practice, Vanderbilt University Medical Center, Nashville, Tennessee

HSIN-MEI CHEN, PhD, MBA
Assistant Professor of Nursing, Institute for Academic Medicine, Houston Methodist Hospital, Houston, Texas

LADONNA CHRISTY, MSN, RN, CCRN
Nurse Education Specialist II, Center for Professional Excellence, Houston Methodist Hospital, Houston, Texas

JOHNNY DANG, DNP, CRNA
Department of Acute and Continuing Care, University of Texas Health Science Center at Houston, Houston, Texas

SARAH DAVIS, DNP, AGACNP, FNP
Department of Advanced Practice, Vanderbilt University Medical Center, Nashville, Tennessee

MINDY FRENCH, BSN, MSN, ACNP-BC
Department of Anesthesiology and Perioperative Medicine, Oregon Health and Science University, Portland, Oregon

SHANNAN K. HAMLIN, PhD, RN, ACNP-BC, AGACNP-BC, CCRN NE-BC
Director, Center for Professional Excellence, Assistant Professor of Nursing, Institute for Academic Medicine, Houston Methodist Hospital, Houston, Texas

BRADLEY R. HARRELL, DNP, APRN, ACNP-BC
Assistant Professor, Loewenberg College of Nursing, University of Memphis, Memphis, Tennessee; International Nurse Member/Contributor, Nursing Management Guidelines Workgroup for Intra-Abdominal Hypertension and Abdominal Compartment Syndrome, WSACS - The Abdominal Compartment Society, Richmond, Virginia

CRAIG HUTTO, BSN, MSN, AGACNP-BC
Department of Anesthesiology and Perioperative Medicine, Oregon Health and Science University, Portland, Oregon

ROSE MILANO, RN, BSN, MS, DNP, ACNP-BC
Assistant Professor, Adult-Gerontology Acute Care Nurse Practitioner Program, School of Nursing, Trauma Nurse Practitioner/Assistant Professor, School of Medicine, Oregon Health and Science University, Portland, Oregon

ROBIN K. MILLER, MSN, ACNP-BC, CHFN
Nurse Practitioner, Heart Failure and Transplant, Knight Cardiovascular Institute; Professor, Adult-Gerontology Acute Care Nurse Practitioner Program, Oregon Health and Science University, Portland, Oregon

SARAH MILLER, PhD, RN
Associate Professor, Medical University of South Carolina, College of Nursing, Charleston, South Carolina

BENJAMIN STUART SCHULTZE, PhD, MSN, MEd
Assistant Professor of Nursing, Oregon Health & Science University School of Nursing, Adult-Gerontlogy Acute Care Nurse Practitioner Program, Portland, Oregon

AMANDA N. SQUIERS, DNP, APRN, ANP-BC, GNP-BC
Clinical Assistant Professor, Oregon Health and Science University School of Nursing; Department of Urologic Surgery, Clinical Instructor, Oregon Health and Science University School of Medicine, Portland, Oregon

PENELOPE Z. STRAUSS, PhD, MSN, CRNA
Independent Consultant, Houston, Texas

NATHANIEL THORNTON, MN, AGACNP-BC
Doctor of Nursing Practice Student, Oregon Health and Science University School of Nursing, Portland, Oregon

KARLEENA TWITCHELL, MN, APRN
Division of Cardiac and Surgical Subspecialty Critical Care, Department of Anesthesiology, Instructor of Anesthesiology, Oregon Health and Science University School of Medicine, Portland, Oregon

BRIANA WITHERSPOON, DNP, APRN, ACNP
Assistant Director of Advanced Practice, Neuroscience, Neuroscience Critical Care Nurse Practitioner, Assistant in Critical Care, Departments of Anesthesiology and Advanced Practice, Vanderbilt University Medical Center, Nashville, Tennessee

Contents

The resuscitation of an adult trauma patient has been researched and written about for the past century. Throughout those discussions, 2 major controversies persist when discussing resuscitation methods: (1) the ideal choice of fluid type to use during the initial resuscitation period, and (2) the ideal fluid volume to infuse during the initial resuscitation period. This article presents a brief historical perspective of fluids used during a trauma resuscitation, along with the latest research findings as they relate to the 2 stated issues.

Patients with increased intracranial pressure generally require pharmacologic therapies and often more definitive treatments, such as surgical intervention. The overall goal of these interventions is to maintain or re-establish adequate cerebral blood flow and prevent herniation. Regardless of the cause of increased intracranial pressure, osmotherapy is considered the mainstay of medical therapy, and should be administered as soon as possible. This article reviews the history of hyperosmolar and hypertonic therapies, the Monro-Kellie hypothesis, and types of cerebral edema. Pharmacologic properties, clinical applications, complications, recommended monitoring during therapy, and risks versus benefits are also discussed.

Chronic heart failure is a chronic condition that is associated with increased health care expenditures and high rates of morbidity and mortality. Mainstay in heart failure management has been the prescription of a fluid restriction. The purpose of this article is to review the available evidence for fluid restriction in chronic heart failure patients.

Ultrasonography is a first-line diagnostic tool when evaluating volume status in the critical care patient population. Ultrasonography leads to a prompt diagnosis and more appropriate management plan, while decreasing health care costs, time to diagnosis, hospital length of stay, time to definitive operation, and mortality. It is recommended that critical care providers treating critically ill patients be skilled and competent in critical care ultrasonography. As the critical care population and the shortage of critical care physicians increases, advanced practice providers are becoming more prevalent in critical care areas and should be competent in this skill as well.

Many urologic reconstructive techniques involve the use of autologous bowel for urinary diversion and bladder augmentation. The resection of bowel and its reimplantation into the urinary system often comes with a variety of metabolic and electrolyte derangements, depending on the type of bowel used and the quantity of urine it is exposed to in its final anatomic position. Clinicians should be aware of these potential complications due to the serious consequences that may result from uncorrected electrolyte disturbances. This article reviews the common electrolyte complications related to both bowel resection and the interposition of bowel within the urinary tract.

The microcirculation is responsible for blood flow regulation and red blood cell distribution throughout individual organs. Patients with circulatory shock have acute failure of the cardiovascular system in which there is insufficient delivery of oxygen to meet metabolic tissue requirements. All subtypes of shock pathophysiology have a hypovolemic component. Fluid resuscitation guided by systemic hemodynamic end points is a common intervention. Evidence shows that microcirculatory shock persists even after optimization of macrocirculatory hemodynamics. The ability for nurses to assess the microcirculation at the bedside in real-time during fluid resuscitation could lead to improved algorithms designed to resuscitate the microcirculation.

Overall, there is a lack of randomized controlled trials examining the correlation between fluid volume delivery and outcomes in postoperative lung transplant patients. However, using thoracic surgery patients as a guide, the evidence suggests that hypervolemia correlates with pulmonary edema and should be avoided in lung transplant patients. However, it is recognized that patients with hemodynamic instability may require volume for attenuation of this situation, but it can likely be mitigated with the use of inotropic medication to maintain adequate perfusion and avoid the development of edema.

Tumor lysis syndrome (TLS) is a life-threatening disorder that is an oncologic emergency. Risk factors for TLS are well-known, but the current literature shows case descriptions of unexpected acute TLS. Solid tumors and untreated hematologic tumors can lyse under various circumstances in children and adults. International guidelines and recommendations, including the early involvement of the critical care team, have been put forward to help clinicians properly manage the syndrome. Advanced practice nurses may be in the position of triaging and initiating treatment of patients with TLS, and need a thorough understanding of the syndrome and its treatment.

Dysnatremia is a common finding in the intensive care unit (ICU) and may be a predictor for mortality and poor clinical outcomes. Depending on the time of onset (ie, on admission vs later in the ICU stay), the incidence of dysnatremias in critically ill patients ranges from 6.9% to 15%, respectively. The symptoms of sodium derangement and their effect on brain physiology make early recognition and correction paramount in the neurologic ICU. Hyponatremia in brain injured patients can lead to life-threatening conditions such as seizures and may worsen cerebral edema and contribute to alterations in intracranial pressure.

Fluid resuscitation is a primary concern of nurse clinicians. Excessive resuscitation with crystalloids places patients at particular risk for many subsequent complications that carry associated increases in mortality and morbidity. Intra-abdominal hypertension and abdominal compartment syndrome are deadly complications of third spacing and capillary leak that occur secondary to excessive fluid resuscitation. Careful consideration is necessary when achieving fluid balance in acutely ill patients, including reducing the use of crystalloids, implementing damage control resuscitation, and establishing measurable resuscitation endpoints. Nurse clinicians are capable of reducing mortality in intra-abdominal hypertension and abdominal compartment syndrome patients by incorporating the latest evidence in fluid resuscitation techniques.

NURSING CLINICS OF NORTH AMERICA

Foreword

I Sing the Body Electric: Where It All Begins

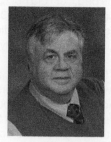

Stephen D. Krau, PhD, RN, CNE
Consulting Editor

> *I sing the body electric.*
> —*Walt Whitman, Leaves of Grass, 1855*

One of the least understood phenomena in our profession is the measurement and empirics related to fluid and electrolytes of the human body. There are on-going debates and discussions about balances, accurate methods of measurement, and the importance of fluid and electrolyte balance. When one considers the human body in its most fundamental form, even more simplistic than the cellular level, one must consider electrolytes and their relationship to body fluids. It is not feasible to consider one without the other. Our basic existence is the result of fluids, and their relationships to the atomic particles that are electrically charged that circulate in our being and in our world. As Walt Whitman so eloquently described, "I sing the body electric."

We are connected to the world through many of the same elements thought to exist at the beginning of time. Humans arrived relatively late on the scene, billions of years from what many scientists describe as the inception of earth. Because billions is a very abstract concept, an understanding of the timing of man can best be understood through an analogy of a calendar year. If one considers the beginning of earth as the start of a new year, such as 00:01 AM on January 1, then reflects on the remaining months, days, hours, and minutes throughout that year, it is more comprehensible. Considering a whole calendar year, humans arrived on the scene at 11:45 PM on December 31 of that year. So within the scope of a year, we have been on this planet for only 15 minutes! And we emerged from the same fluids and elements that existed more than likely since the beginning.

Fluid and electrolyte balance is one of the key factors in the maintenance of homeostasis and is essential in maintaining and protecting cellular function as well as acid-base balance and tissue perfusion. Electrolyte balance is contingent on many intricate

Nurs Clin N Am 52 (2017) ix–x
http://dx.doi.org/10.1016/j.cnur.2017.03.002
0029-6465/17/© 2017 Published by Elsevier Inc.

factors beyond the actual electrolyte itself. Hormonal influences, fluid balance, and many disease processes impact this delicate, but essential balance.

Fluid balances and measurements remain a major concern for health care providers and systems. The National Confidential Enquiry into Perioperative Deaths (NCEPOD) and the National Patient Safety Agency identify that despite efforts earlier this century, inadequacies in measurement and fluid balance charts are low priorities in many settings.[1] Ambiguous notations, such as "voided in toilet," "wet the bed," or "did not capture," are commonly recorded as opposed to actual volumes passed. In 1999, NCEPOD recommended that "fluid management be given the same status as medication prescribing."[1] Many barriers remain to the management of fluids and electrolytes in the acute care setting.

Although efforts are being made to be more precise about fluid measurement, it is still vague and not always a priority, and the importance is not well understood. Nurses are *charged* with learning as much as they can about fluid and electrolytes, although the topics may seem daunting. We have made so many strides in other areas, yet this basic and most foundational marvel eludes many of us. But then, I guess one could argue, "Hey, we have only had 15 minutes!"

Stephen D. Krau, PhD, RN, CNE
School of Nursing
Vanderbilt University
461 21st Avenue South
Nashville, TN 37240, USA

E-mail address:
sbluefountain@aol.com

REFERENCE

1. McGloin S. The ins and outs of fluid balance in the acutely ill patient. Br J Nurs 2015;24(1):14–8.

Preface

Current Issues in Fluid and Electrolyte Management

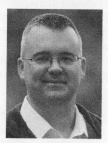

Joshua Squiers, PhD, ACNP-BC, AGACNP-BC, FCCM
Editor

Excellence is achieved by the mastery of the fundamentals.

—Vince Lombardi

There is nothing more fundamental to the practice of critical care nursing than an understanding of the function and potential derangements of our homeostatic fluids and electrolytes. The history of bodily fluids and their associated electrolytes is long and somewhat arduous.

The role of bodily fluids in human physiology has been recognized since ancient times. Previous works focusing on the circulatory system note that early man recognized that blood was a bodily fluid required for sustaining life. Ancient man knew that compression of the carotids led to unconsciousness, that bleeding led to death, and that applying pressure to bleeding wounds prevented death on the battlefield.[1] Between 400 and 200 BCE, Greek philosophers applied humoral theory to medicine and further recognized the role of blood and other bodily fluids, including yellow bile, black bile, and phlegm, on health and disease. The role of bodily fluids has been recognized since early man, but the role of electrolytes has been a more recent advance.

The initial understanding of electrolytes developed the work of Svante Arrhenius (1859-1927), a Swedish-born chemist whose doctoral dissertation "Investigations on the galvanic conductivity of electrolytes" solidified the definition of electrolytes and provided a framework for understanding their behavior in water. This work developed into the electrolytic dissociation theory that is currently used throughout modern science and that won him the Nobel Prize in Chemistry in 1903. While the majority of his work focused on the physical chemistry of electrolytes, he provided some of the initial work around the role of electrolytes in digestion and absorption.[2] His scientific work provides much of the foundation for modern electrolyte physiology and clinical care.

Nurs Clin N Am 52 (2017) xi–xii
http://dx.doi.org/10.1016/j.cnur.2017.03.001
0029-6465/17/© 2017 Published by Elsevier Inc.

Despite a long history of continued research, our understanding of the management of fluid and electrolyte derangements remains in its infancy. Almost all clinicians deal with these clinical issues in some way on a daily basis. The purpose of this issue is to highlight some of the current ongoing discussions surrounding fluid and electrolyte management in the acute care settings. Each of these articles describes a challenging clinical issue related to fluids and electrolytes in a variety of clinical settings, including heart failure, extracorporeal life support, intracranial pressure management, intravascular volume status assessment, and many others. The authors hope that these discussions stimulate further clinical work surrounding these topics and act as a resource for clinicians wanting an updated discussion of current issues.

Ultimately, there is nothing more fundamental than fluids and electrolytes in clinical care, and we hope this issue will assist clinicians in refining their views on these important topics.

Joshua Squiers, PhD, ACNP-BC, AGACNP-BC, FCCM
OHSU School of Nursing
OHSU School of Medicine
Division of Cardiac and
Surgical Subspecialty Critical Care
Department of Anesthesiology and
Perioperative Medicine
Mail Code: SN-6S
3455 SW US Veterans Hospital Road
Portland, OR 97239-2941, USA

E-mail address:
squiers@ohsu.edu

REFERENCES

1. Nobelprize.org. Svante Arrhenius—biographical. Nobel Media AB 2014. Available at: http://www.nobelprize.org/nobel_prizes/chemistry/laureates/1903/arrhenius-bio.html. Accessed August 8, 2016.
2. Garrison F. An outline of the history of the circulatory system. Bull N Y Acad Med 1931;7(10):781–806.

Fluid Resuscitation of the Adult Trauma Patient

Where Have We Been and Where Are We Going?

Rose Milano, RN, BSN, MS, DNP, ACNP-BC

KEYWORDS

• Resuscitation • Trauma • Fluids • Crystalloids • Colloids • Blood • Volume

KEY POINTS

• Colloids have fallen out of favor because of the ever-increasing data surrounding complications.

• Conservative volume resuscitation is becoming the new standard.

• There is an abundance of current research investigating the optimal use of blood products during trauma resuscitations.

INTRODUCTION

Trauma-related injuries remain the leading cause of death in individuals ages 1 to 44.[1] Uncontrolled hemorrhage is the leading cause of preventable death in the traumatically injured adult, with more than 50% of deaths occurring within the first 12 hours of injury.[2] Managing the high morbidity and mortality of traumatic hemorrhage encompasses stopping the bleeding, possible surgical intervention, fluid resuscitation, and blood transfusion therapy.[3] Trauma researchers have long sought to identify the ideal fluid replacement therapy to be used during initial resuscitation efforts. This article provides a brief historical perspective of fluid resuscitation, explores the advantages and disadvantages of the 3 most common fluids used during initial resuscitation efforts (crystalloids, colloids, and blood products), and presents concise discussion points regarding the aggressive versus controlled volume resuscitation debate.

OVERVIEW OF RESUSCITATION FLUID THERAPY

Researchers have recommended that resuscitative fluid therapy should be thought of as any other medications, and described using the 4Ds when providing fluid therapy (Table 1).[4] A hypotensive adult patient who has suffered a traumatic injury is believed

Adult-Gerontology Acute Care Nurse Practitioner Program, Division of Trauma, Critical Care and Acute Care Surgery, Department of Surgery, School of Nursing, School of Medicine, Oregon Health and Science University, 3455 Southwest US Veterans Hospital Road, Portland, OR 97239, USA
E-mail address: milano@ohsu.edu

Nurs Clin N Am 52 (2017) 237–247
http://dx.doi.org/10.1016/j.cnur.2017.01.001
0029-6465/17/© 2017 Elsevier Inc. All rights reserved.

Table 1
Identification and explanation of the 4 Ds

Identification of D	Explanation of D
Drug	Providing the right fluid for the right patient at the right time, taking into consideration patient risk factors, such as kidney function, cardiac status, source control, fluid balance, and potential for capillary leak.
Dose	Providing the right dose and the right speed of infusion based on the pharmacokinetics, pharmacodynamics, and toxicity profile of the fluid being infused.
Duration	Providing the fluids for only as long as needed and not continuing treatment once a positive patient response has been achieved.
De-escalation	Withdrawing or withholding fluids when they are no longer needed.

Data from Malbrain ML, Van Regenmortel N, Owczuk R. It is time to consider the four D's of fluid management. Anaesthesiol Intensive Ther 2015;47:s1–5.

to be in hemorrhagic shock until proven otherwise. This shock state is a major risk factor for multiple organ dysfunction and mortality.[5] Although the use of intravenous fluids is a common intervention used during trauma resuscitation, the choice of which fluid is best to replace the fluid losses has been a long-standing controversy. Four major goals for the initial resuscitation of an adult trauma patient have been identified:

1. To restore the loss of circulating intravascular volume
2. To ensure adequate delivery of oxygen to the vital organs
3. To decrease the risk of resuscitation complications
4. To enhance the ability to form blood clots at the site of active bleeding[6]

Crystalloids are composed of fluids and electrolytes that when administered increase intravascular volume and decrease plasma oncotic pressure. They are predominately sodium-containing solutions that freely diffuse between the intravascular and interstitial fluid compartments. The primary result of intravenously infusing a crystalloid solution is the expansion of the interstitial, not the plasma, volume. If 1 L of crystalloid is infused, it is estimated that 25% (or 250 mL) will expand the plasma volume, whereas 75% (or 750 mL) will expand the interstitial fluid volume.[7]

Colloids act differently in that their molecular structure contains larger molecules that do not pass freely between the plasma and interstitial spaces. This results in a preservation of oncotic pressure, an increase in plasma volume by holding water within the vascular compartment when colloids are infused intravenously.[7(p227)] Last, the administration of whole blood during the initial phase of the resuscitation of a trauma patient was the original fluid of choice before the development of synthetic fluids. Blood components typically have been given when the need to address laboratory test deficiencies has been identified.[5(p1407)] It has been historically advocated that the best product to provide to a patient in shock is the product that the patient has lost. For instance, if the patient has suffered significant blood loss, as in hemorrhagic shock, then blood should be given. If a patient has lost nonblood fluid volume, as in dehydration, then crystalloids should be given.[8] With the variety of choices available these days, the ideal fluid to resuscitate an adult trauma patient has been described as one that would (1) produce a predictable and sustainable increase in intravascular volume, (2) have a chemical make up as close as possible to extracellular fluid, (3) be metabolized and excreted without excess accumulation in tissues, (4) not produce adverse metabolic or systemic effects, and (5) be cost-effective while improving patient outcomes.[9] Unfortunately, there is no current fluid available that addresses all of these recommendations successfully. Fluids used during resuscitation are broadly categorized as blood, crystalloids, and colloids (**Fig. 1**). Each type of replacement fluid has both advantages and disadvantages.

ADVANCED TRAUMA LIFE SUPPORT FLUID RESUSCITATION RECOMMENDATIONS

Current Advanced Trauma Life Support (ATLS) guidelines recommend packed red blood cell transfusions for the acute adult trauma patient who does not respond/minimally responds or transiently responds to an initial intravenous crystalloid bolus of 1 to 2 L lactated Ringer's solution.[10] The ATLS guidelines define nonresponders/minimal responders as those patients who have no improvement or minimal improvement in their vital signs, plus they demonstrate no other signs of adequate organ/tissue perfusion after the initial fluid bolus. Transient responders are defined as those patients who have an initial improvement in their vital signs that does not last and they again become hypotensive and tachycardic. These ATLS guidelines recommend the following on how to monitor for adequate organ/tissue perfusion in response to an initial fluid bolus given during resuscitation: (1) a patient who does not produce 0.5 mg/kg per hour of urine output is noted to be underresuscitated, and (2) serial monitoring of lactic acid levels, a by-product of anaerobic metabolism caused by inadequate tissue perfusion, also provides an indication of how well the patient has been resuscitated.

Blood

The first recorded blood transfusion was not given for hemorrhage but was given to Pope Innocent VIII in 1490, who was dying of old age. To treat this patient, his physician injected the Pope with blood from 3 healthy young men, believing this would rejuvenate his ailing body. It was reported that not only did the Pope die, the 3 young men also perished, causing the physician to flee his country.[11] The use of whole blood transfusions continued until the 1970s, with the emergence of blood component

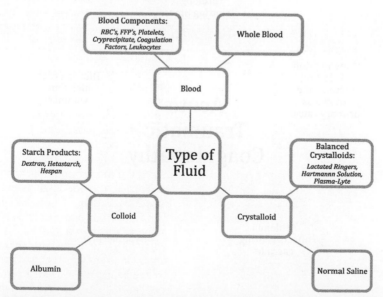

Fig. 1. Categories of resuscitation fluids. FFP, fresh frozen plasma; RBC, red blood cell.

infusion therapy in which red blood cells, platelets, and plasma are infused separately or in varying combinations in place of whole blood. Although there was no supportive research demonstrating equal efficacy in transfusing whole blood versus its separate components, this quickly became the standard of practice throughout the country.[8(p3)] An impaired coagulation state rapidly ensues with the combination of tissue injury and systemic hypoperfusion when a severe traumatic injury is sustained. **Fig. 2** identifies multiple drivers that predispose the injured trauma patient to developing acute traumatic coagulopathy.[12]

This endogenous traumatic coagulopathy has been noted to increase mortality threefold to sixfold. Researchers have identified a web-type membrane, the glycocalyx layer, within the endothelium that plays a vital role in maintaining the membrane permeability of the endothelial vascular bed.[9(p1244)] Researchers also have found that transfusing with plasma during hypovolemic resuscitation preserves this glycocalyx layer better than other resuscitation fluid options.[13] They have documented that the coagulopathy experienced by individuals with major traumatic injuries is by driven dozens, possibly hundreds, of molecules and mediators that affect clotting factors even before substantial fluid losses have been observed.[13(p4)] This research highlights the importance of early recognition and prompt treatment for the survival of the traumatically injured adult. Massive transfusion is required for many of these critically injured patients, which is defined as administration of more than 10 units of blood within a 24-hour period, or more than 5 units of blood within the first 4 hours.[14] Although blood components have virtually replaced the practice of transfusing whole blood during trauma resuscitation, there is research from the military that demonstrates whole blood is more efficient than blood component transfusions in correcting acute

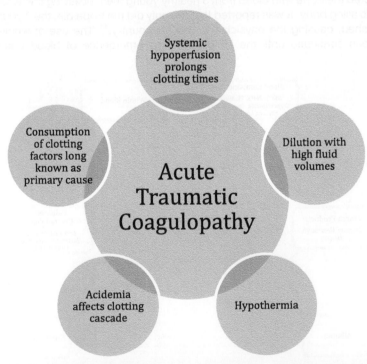

Fig. 2. Drivers predisposing trauma patients to developing acute traumatic coagulopathy.

coagulopathies and restoring hemostasis in war victims who are in shock. They have also demonstrated that whole blood minimizes the risk of known harmful effects of using old stored packed red blood cells.[14(p89)] A summary of major advantages and disadvantages/limitations of using blood during trauma resuscitation are found in **Table 2**.

Crystalloids

In 1832, Robert Lewins described how he used intravenous injections of a saline solution to treat the effects of dehydration suffered during the cholera pandemic in Scotland.[9(p1234)] The use of a variety of different concentrated saline solutions continued until the addition by Sidney Ringer in 1883 of what has become known as Ringer's solution, and in 1932 with the development of the Hartmann solution by Alexis Hartmann. Hartmann, who was a practicing pediatrician treating the dehydration noted in his patients with gastroenteritis, added a buffer (lactate) to the Ringer's solution and invented what we now call lactated Ringer's solution, or Hartmann solution.[21,22]

Crystalloid solutions are divided into 2 main categories: 0.9% normal saline and balanced (lactated Ringer's, Hartmann, and Plasma-Lyte) solutions.[21(p1541)] Although the use of these solutions had initially been interchangeable, it has been demonstrated there is not only a variance in their chemical makeup (**Table 3**), but also an increasing amount of evidence connecting a significant side-effect profile with the use infusion of normal saline.[21(pp1541–1542),22(pp207,231),23] Normal saline has a 50% higher concentration of chloride than plasma, which when infused rapidly and in large volumes has been found to cause hyperchloremic metabolic acidosis, confusing providers when interpreting the underlying cause of the acid-base disorder to treat increase their interventions in an attempt to correct the pH, which in turn leads to increased patient length of stay.[21(p1541)] Others have noted that this hyperchloremia increases renal vascular resistance, which leads to decreased blood flow to the kidneys causing acute kidney injury.[22(p213)] A link has been identified between the resultant hyperchloremic acidosis and increased extravascular lung water and coagulopathy.[23(p14)] It also has been noted that normal saline with a lower concentration of magnesium, when compared

Table 2
Advantages/disadvantages of blood administration

Advantages of Blood Administration	Disadvantages/Limitations of Blood Administration
Increase in Hgb/Hct: 1 unit RBCs estimated to raise Hgb/Hct @1 g/dL and 3%, respectively	Prolonged storage of RBCs before transfusion shown to impair tissue oxygenation
Increased oxygen delivery with RBCs	No/limited improvement in oxygen extraction with RBCs
Plasma contains high concentrations of protease inhibitors, which regulate fibrinolysis and enhance return of hemostasis	Potential complications include nonhemolytic fever, urticaria-transmitted infections, anaphylaxis/anaphylactic shock, acute lung injury, transfusion errors, acute to fatal hemolytic reaction
RBC administration accelerates the onset of clot formation	Limited supporting research equating positive patient outcomes between whole blood transfusions vs combined blood component transfusion therapies
Plasma preserves endothelial glycocalyx layer of vascular bed	Limited availability of whole blood, blood components

Abbreviations: Hgb/Hct, hemoglobin/hematocrit; RBC, red blood cell.
Data from Refs.[7,15–20]

Table 3
Composition of commonly used crystalloid solutions

| | Specific Crystalloid Solution Configuration | | | | | |
	Osmolarity	Sodium	Potassium	Chloride	Calcium	Lactate
Saline	308	154	X	154	X	X
Ringer's lactate	280	130	4.0	109	1.5	28
Hartmann solution	277	131	5.4	112	1.8	28
Plasma-Lyte	294	140	5.0	98	X	X

X indicates 0 or negligent.
Data from Myburgh JA, Mythen MG. Resuscitation fluids. N Engl J Med 2013;369(13):1243–51.

with Plasma-Lyte, adds an additional cost to the patient and institution in magnesium-replacement therapy.[24] This and other mounting evidence[25–27] has led many providers to choose alternative infusing crystalloid solutions over normal saline. Yet, many practitioners continue to support the use of normal saline, basing their argument on limited evidence reporting the complications may not translate into clinically significant adverse effects on patient outcomes.[28–31]

A summary of major advantages and disadvantages/limitations of using normal saline versus balanced solutions during trauma resuscitation are summarized in **Table 4**.

Table 4
Comparisons of major advantages and disadvantages/limitations of crystalloid solution administration

Advantages of Crystalloid Solution Administration		Disadvantages/Limitations of Crystalloid Solution Administration	
Lactated Ringer's, Hartmann, Plasma-Lyte	0.9% Normal Saline	Lactated Ringer's, Hartmann, Plasma-Lyte	0.9% Normal Saline
Widely available Cost equivalent to all crystalloids	Widely available Cost equivalent to all crystalloids	Increased lactate levels → shown to not be associated with clinical significance	Hyperchloremic metabolic acidosis
Less expensive than colloids	Less expensive than colloids	Increased mortality in traumatic brain injury when compared with normal saline	Decreased renal blood flow, glomerular filtration rate, compromising renal tissue perfusion → increased risk of acute kidney injury
No problem with hypomagnesemia	Able to infuse with blood transfusions	Does not replace clotting factors	Does not replace clotting factors
Increased renal tissue perfusion		Unable to infuse with blood transfusions	Increased extravascular lung water → respiratory complications
			Resultant hypomagnesemia

Data from Refs.[21–32]

Colloids

The care of military personnel during wartime has consistently provided valuable information that has become vital in caring for the civilian population. During World War I, military physicians noted 2 significant details. When a patient had suffered the loss of a significant volume of blood, the use of intravenous saline solutions to treat hemorrhagic shock was inadequate, and although providing blood would be optimal for these patients, there was no blood available for transfusions on the battlefield. The physicians knew they needed a fluid to improve survival of these patients while being transported off the battlefield to the medical unit where they could be given optimal treatment, and the development of colloid solutions emerged. During World War II, the use of human albumin became readily available and standard practice to treat burn patients from the Pearl Harbor attack. Synthetic albumin products have since been developed because of the high cost of fractionating human albumin.[22(pp210-212)]

Randomized controlled trials (RCTs) comparing colloids with crystalloids during fluid resuscitation of critically ill patients were reviewed and results reported in 2013 by The Cochrane Collaboration. They sought to answer the question if colloids were more effective than crystalloids in decreasing mortality in the critically ill patient. They searched multiple databases from 1946 through 2012, including critically ill patients with burns or trauma, and those undergoing surgery or any other conditions that developed into critical illness, such as sepsis. The fluids they researched included multiple types of colloids (including albumin, dextran, hydroxyethyl starches, and modified gelatins) plus isotonic and hypertonic crystalloids. The only outcome measure investigated was the death of the patient. The investigators concluded on completing their review that there was no RCT evidence that colloids decreased mortality in trauma, burns, or after surgery when compared with crystalloid solutions. In addition, they reported that some studies found that hydroxyethyl may actually increase mortality. Finally, their recommendation was that because there was no difference in mortality, and colloids were a more expensive option, that colloids were not a practical fluid solution option.[33] In addition, researchers found that albumin as a resuscitation fluid carried a higher mortality rate than crystalloids when caring for the patient with traumatic brain injury; thus, colloid infusions are not recommended for these patients.[34]

AGGRESSIVE/HIGH-VOLUME VERSUS CONTROLLED-VOLUME RESUSCITATION

Multiple adverse effects in almost every physiologic system throughout the body have been reported when a critically ill patient becomes fluid overloaded. Cerebral edema, pulmonary edema, pleural effusions, myocardial overload, pericardial effusions, gastrointestinal edema, hepatic congestion/ascites, renal vascular edema, tissue edema, and impaired lymphatic drainage with abnormal microcirculation are all possible when a patient has been overburdened with fluid during a resuscitation while attempting to restore hemostasis.[35] As early as 1918, it was recognized that administering massive amounts of intravenous fluids before the bleeding was controlled actually led to increased bleeding.[36]

Understanding that shock and poor tissue perfusion are strong independent risk factors for poor patient outcomes in the traumatically injured patient, for decades the standard of practice in restoring the circulating volume, and sustaining tissue and vital organ perfusion during resuscitation was to provide large volumes of intravenous fluid replacement. As early as 1994, this practice came under scrutiny by researchers who found that providing large volumes of fluids before controlling bleeding was actually detrimental to the patient.[37] Although researchers in 1994 did not propose a theory as to how rapid fluid resuscitation caused harmful effects in their patient population, they did identify that patients who received the standard rapid fluid infusion experienced a greater amount of adult respiratory syndrome, acute renal failure, sepsis, coagulopathies, wound infections, and pneumonia when compared with patients who received a delayed fluid resuscitation.

Subsequently, over the years more and more researchers have investigated this phenomenon and reinforced the knowledge that controlled resuscitation actually improved patient survival. It is hypothesized that aggressive fluid administration causes a dilution of coagulation factors and hyperfibrinolysis, likely by the release of tissue plasminogen activator from damaged tissues, leading to the destruction of newly formed clots and intensifying the hemorrhagic state.[37,38] A systematic review of the literature (looking at fluid overload, deresuscitation, and outcomes in critically ill patients) concluded that restrictive fluid management was associated with a lower incidence of intra-abdominal hypertension and a lower mortality rate when compared with patients who were given fluids more liberally.[39] It has also been reported that

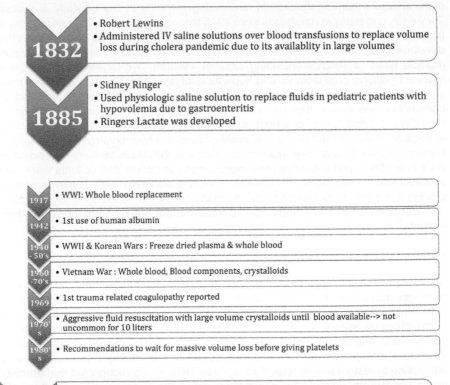

1832
- Robert Lewins
- Administered IV saline solutions over blood transfusions to replace volume loss during cholera pandemic due to its availablity in large volumes

1885
- Sidney Ringer
- Used physiologic saline solution to replace fluids in pediatric patients with hypovolemia due to gastroenteritis
- Ringers Lactate was developed

1917 · WWI: Whole blood replacement

1942 · 1st use of human albumin

1940 -50's · WWII & Korean Wars : Freeze dried plasma & whole blood

1960 -70's · Vietnam War : Whole blood, Blood components, crystalloids

1969 · 1st trauma related coagulopathy reported

1970's · Aggressive fluid resuscitation with large volume crystalloids until blood available--> not uncommon for 10 liters

1980's · Recommendations to wait for massive volume loss before giving platelets

2000's
- Aggressive versus controlled volume replacement
- Returning to using of whole blood & blood components during resuscitation
- What is the optimal combination of blood components? RBC:Plasma:Platelets?

Fig. 3. Historical perspective of resuscitation therapies over the years. IV, intravenous; WWI, World War I; WWII, World War II. (*Data from* Holcomb J. Resuscitation history. Lecture presented: 27th Annual Northwest States Trauma Conference. Bend (OR), May 5, 2016.)

once a critically injured trauma patient regained a normotensive state and their intravenous fluid volume was decreased, they had required less ventilator support and had a shorter length of stay in the intensive care unit.[40] Although the debate over aggressive versus controlled fluid resuscitation continues, more and more research is highlighting adverse effects of aggressive fluid administration and the need for more cautious fluid administration during resuscitation of the critically ill trauma patient.

SUMMARY

Stabilizing an acutely injured hypovolemic trauma patient requires aggressive treatment to stop the bleeding and replace the lost fluid volume while restoring perfusion to vital organs and tissues. As discussed in this article, the controversy over the selection of optimal resuscitation fluids continues. Although some researchers advocate normal saline, others recommend a more balanced solution, such as lactated Ringer's solution. The use of colloids, shown to have no added benefits and many negative effects, has fallen out of favor. In addition, investigators are reporting a return to a practice that had faded with time. It is once again being demonstrated that the sooner a traumatically injured patient is administered blood and its components, the chance of surviving traumatic injuries increases. There is an abundance of current research investigating the optimal use of blood products during trauma resuscitations, which appears to be a cyclical pattern when looking at the history of fluid resuscitation (**Fig. 3**). In conclusion, with the ongoing controversies outlined in this article, it is incumbent on all providers caring for adult trauma patients to remain up to date on the latest research so as to provide the highest quality patient care.

REFERENCES

1. Injury Prevention and Control: Data Statistics. 2013. Available at: http://www.cdc. gov/injury/wisqars/overview/key_data.html. Accessed November 8, 2016.
2. MacLeod JB, Cohn SM, Johnson EW, et al. Trauma deaths in the first hour: are they all unsalvageable? Am J Surg 2007;193:195–9.
3. Curry N, Hopewell S, Doree C, et al. The acute management of trauma hemorrhage: a systematic review of randomized controlled trials. Crit Care 2011; 15:R92.
4. Malbrain ML, Van Regenmortel N, Owczuk R. It is time to consider the four D's of fluid resuscitation. Anaesthesiol Intensive Ther 2015;47:s1–5.
5. Kobayashi L, Costantini TW, Coimbra R. Hypovolemic shock. Surg Clin North Am 2012;92:1403–23.
6. Butler FK, Holcomb JB, Schreiber MA, et al. Fluid resuscitation for hemorrhagic shock in tactical combat casualty care. J Spec Operations Med 2014;14(3): 13–37.
7. Marino P. The ICU book. 4th edition. Philadelphia: Wolters Kluwer Health; 2014. p. 217–34.
8. McSwain NE, Champion HR, Fabian TC, et al. State of the art of fluid resuscitation 2010: prehospital and immediate transition to the hospital. J Trauma 2011;70(5): S2–10.
9. Myburgh JA, Mythen MG. Resuscitation fluids. N Engl J Med 2013;369(13): 1243–51.
10. Rotondo MF, Fildes J. Advanced trauma life support: student course manual. 9th edition. Chicago: American College Surgeons; 2012.
11. Wood CS. A short history of blood transfusion. Transfusion 1967;7(4):299–300.

12. Brohl K, Cohen MJ, Davenport RA. Acute coagulopathy of trauma: mechanism, identification and effect. Curr Opin Crit Care 2007;13:680–5.
13. Dutton RP. Management of traumatic haemorrhage—the US perspective. Ansethesia 2015;70(1):108–13.
14. McGrath C. Blood transfusion strategies for hemostatic resuscitation in massive trauma. Nurs Clin North Am 2016;51:83–93.
15. Marik PE, Corwin HL. Efficacy of red blood cell transfusion in the critically ill: a systematic review of literature. Crit Care Med 2008;36:2667–74.
16. Fuller BM, Gajera M, Schorr C. Transfusion of packed red blood cells is not associated with improved central venous oxygenation saturation or organ function in patients with septic shock. J Emerg Med 2012;43:593–8.
17. Kiraly LN, Underwood S, Differding JA, et al. Transfusion of aged packed red blood cells results in decreased tissue oxygenation in critically ill trauma patients. J Trauma 2009;67(1):29–32.
18. Moore HB, Moore EE, Morton AP, et al. Shock induced systemic hyperfibrinolysis is attenuated by plasma first resuscitation. J Trauma 2015;79(6):897–904.
19. Spoerke NJ, Van PY, Differding JA, et al. Red blood cells accelerate the onset of clot formation in polytrauma and hemorrhagic shock. J Trauma 2010;69(5):1054–9.
20. Strandenes G, Cap AP, Cacic D, et al. Blood far forward: a whole blood research and training program for austere environments. Transfusion 2013;53(S1):124S–30S.
21. Semler MW, Rice TW. Saline is not the first choice for crystalloid resuscitation fluids. Crit Care Med 2016;44(8):1541–4.
22. Kampmeier T, Rehberg S. Evolution of fluid therapy. Best Pract Res Clin Anesthesiol 2014;28:207–16.
23. Schreiber MA. The use of normal saline for resuscitation in trauma. J Trauma 2011;70(5):S13–4.
24. Smith CA, Duby JJ, Utter GH, et al. Cost-minimization analysis of two fluids products for resuscitation of critically ill trauma patients. Am J Health Syst Pharm 2014;71:470–5.
25. Smith CA, Gosselin RC, Utter GH, et al. Does saline resuscitation affect mechanisms of coagulopathy in critically ill trauma patients? An exploratory analysis. Blood Coagul Fibrinolysis 2015;26:250–4.
26. Kiraly LN, Differding JA, Enomoto M, et al. Resuscitation with normal saline [NS] vs. lactated Ringers [LR] modulates hypercoagulability and leads to increased blood loss in an uncontrolled hemorrhagic shock swine model. J Trauma 2006;61(1):57–65.
27. Yunos NM, Bell R, Glassford N, et al. Chloride-liberal vs. chloride-restrictive intravenous fluids administration and acute kidney injury: an extended analysis. Intensive Care Med 2015;41:257–64.
28. Young P. Saline is the solution for crystalloid resuscitation. Crit Care Med 2016;44(8):1538–40.
29. Yunos NM, Bellomo R, Story D, et al. Bench-to-bedside review: chloride in critical illness. Crit Care 2010;14:226.
30. Raghunathan K, Shaw A, Nathanson B, et al. Association between the choice of IV crystalloid and in-hospital mortality among critically ill adults with sepsis. Crit Care Med 2014;42:1585–91.
31. Shaw AD, Schermer CR, Lobo DN, et al. Impact of intravenous fluid composition on outcomes in patients with systemic inflammatory response syndrome. Crit Care 2015;19:334.

32. Rowell SE, Fair KA, Barbosa RR, et al. The impact of pre-hospital administration of lactated Ringer's solution versus normal saline in patients with traumatic brain injury. J Neurotrauma 2016;33:1–6.
33. Perel P, Roberts I, Ker K. Colloids versus crystalloids for fluid resuscitation in critically ill patients: review. Cochrane Database Syst Rev 2013;(2):CD000567.
34. Myburgh J, cooper J, FInfer S, et al. Saline or albumin for fluid resuscitation in patients with traumatic brain injury: the SAFE study investigators. N Engl J Med 2007;357(9):874–84.
35. Ogbu OC, Murphy DJ, Martin GS. How to avoid fluid overload. Curr Opin Crit Care 2015;21:315–21.
36. Cannon WB, Fraser J, Cowell EM. The preventive treatment of wound shock. JAMA 1918;70:618–21.
37. Bickell WH, Wall MJ, Pepe PE, et al. Immediate versus delayed fluid resuscitation for hypotensive patients with penetrating torso injuries. N Engl J Med 1994; 331(17):1105–9.
38. Hampton DA, Fabricant LJ, Differding J, et al. Pre-hospital intravenous fluid is associated with increased survival in trauma patients. J Trauma Acute Care Surg 2013;75(1):s9–15.
39. Schreiber MA, Meier EN, Tisherman SA, et al. A controlled resuscitation strategy is feasible and safe in the hypotensive trauma patient: results of a prospective randomized trial. J Trauma Acute Care Surg 2014;78(4):687–97.
40. Barmparas G, Ara K, Harada M, et al. Decreasing maintenance fluids in normotensive trauma patients may reduce intensive care unit stay and ventilator days. J Crit Care 2016;31:201–5.

The Use of Mannitol and Hypertonic Saline Therapies in Patients with Elevated Intracranial Pressure

A Review of the Evidence

Briana Witherspoon, DNP, APRN, ACNP[a],*, Nathan E. Ashby, MD[b]

KEYWORDS

- Hypertonic saline • Mannitol • Elevated ICP • Intracranial hypertension
- Hyperosmolar therapy

KEY POINTS

- Cerebral edema and elevated intracranial pressure (ICP) are common causes of morbidity and mortality in patients with traumatic brain injuries; intracranial tumors; and cerebral hematomas, infarctions, or hemorrhages.
- Cerebral edema can quickly lead to a downward spiral of worsening intracranial hypertension, cerebral ischemia, and ultimately herniation if not appropriately identified and treated.
- Providing care for patients with increased intracranial pressure generally requires pharmacologic therapies and more definitive treatments, such as surgical intervention. The overall goal of these interventions is to maintain or re-establish adequate cerebral blood flow and prevent herniation.
- Regardless of the cause of increased intracranial pressure, osmotherapy is considered the mainstay of medical therapy, and should be administered as soon as possible.

INTRODUCTION

Cerebral edema and elevated intracranial pressure (ICP) are common causes of morbidity and mortality in patients with traumatic brain injuries (TBI); intracranial tumors; and cerebral hematomas, infarctions, or hemorrhages. Cerebral edema can quickly lead to a downward spiral of worsening intracranial hypertension, cerebral

Disclosure Statement: The authors have nothing to disclose.
[a] Neuroscience, Department of Anesthesiology, Vanderbilt University Medical Center, 1161 21st Avenue South, AA-1214 MCN, Nashville, TN 37232, USA; [b] Department of Anesthesiology, Division of Critical Care, Vanderbilt University Medical Center, 1211 21st Avenue South, MAB 526, Nashville, TN 37212, USA
* Corresponding author.
E-mail address: Briana.m.wickard@vanderbilt.edu

ischemia, and ultimately herniation if not appropriately identified and treated. Although it is estimated that brain death accounts for 2.3% to 11% of all in-hospital deaths, many more patients who develop increased ICP survive with various degrees of cognitive and physical disability.[1] Approximately 1.7 million people in the United States sustain a TBI each year,[2] creating a financial burden of more than $60 billion per year for their ongoing care.[1]

Providing care for patients with increased ICP generally requires pharmacologic therapies and more definitive treatments, such as surgical intervention. The overall goal of these interventions is to maintain or re-establish adequate cerebral blood flow and prevent herniation. Regardless of the cause of increased ICP, osmotherapy is considered the mainstay of medical therapy, and should be administered as soon as possible. Osmotherapy agents temporarily reduce the volume of intracranial contents and allow time for edema to subside or for more definitive treatment, such as a decompressive hemicraniectomy, to be performed.[3]

PATHOPHYSIOLOGY

Given that the cranium is a fixed bony vault, even small increases in the cranial contents cause an increase in ICP. Early work by Monro and Kellie, with contributions by Abercrombie, helped set the stage for current understanding of the interplay between the intracranial contents and the development of elevated ICP.[4] Further work by Magendie, Burrows, Cushing, and others added to the basic understanding of ICP and its formation.[5] The Monro-Kellie hypothesis maintains that an expansion or increase in any one of the intracranial components (brain tissue, intravascular blood, or cerebrospinal fluid [CSF]) must be accompanied by a reduction in one or both of the other components or ICP will subsequently increase.[6,7] In the early stages of intracranial hypertension the CSF is initially forced from the intracranial subarachnoid space and lateral ventricles into the spinal subarachnoid space.[1] As this compensatory mechanism becomes exhausted, blood vessels are compressed and cerebral blood flow is decreased. Once the ICP reaches approximately 50 to 60 mm Hg, it approaches arterial pressure in the vessels of the circle of Willis resulting in global ischemia and ultimately brain death.[1]

Intracranial hypertension is defined as a sustained ICP of greater than 20 mm Hg, with normal ICP ranging between 3 mm Hg and 15 mm Hg.[8] Cerebral perfusion pressure (CPP) is calculated by subtracting the ICP from the mean arterial pressure (MAP). In most healthy adults, cerebral autoregulation maintains a normal CPP between MAPs of 50 mm Hg and 150 mm Hg. If autoregulation is impaired or is outside this range, an increase in MAP also causes an increase in CPP and usually a rise in ICP.[8] Given that the brain parenchyma is composed of nearly 80% water (intracellular and interstitial), its volume is extremely sensitive to fluid shifts.[1] Osmotic therapy uses agents, such as mannitol or hypertonic saline, to create an osmotic gradient across the blood-brain barrier that draws water from the interstitium into the vascular space.[8] (Table 1) The effectiveness of the osmotic agent across the blood-brain barrier can further be explained by using the reflection coefficient of the substance. A value of 0 indicates complete permeability, whereas a value of 1 indicates complete impermeability of the membrane to that substance. The reflection coefficient of sodium against the blood-brain barrier is almost 1, making its efforts at inducing an osmotic gradient between blood and the brain tissue highly effective. Mannitol has a reflection coefficient of 0.9 and is also an effective osmotic agent in reducing brain water content. Ropper[1] points out that in addition to creating an osmotic gradient, mannitol also has the added effect of lowering blood viscosity and causing a reactive

Table 1	
Comparison of mannitol and sodium chloride	
Mannitol	**Sodium Chloride**
Molecular weight: 182.17 g/mol	Molecular weight: 58.45 g/mol
Reflection coefficient: 0.9	Reflection coefficient: 1.0
Sodium content: none	Sodium content
Osmolarity:	• 0.9%: 154 mEq/L
• 20%: 1100 mOsm/L	• 3%: 513 mEq/L
• 25%: 1375 mOsm/L	• 7.5%: 1283 mEq/L
	• 23.4%: 4004 mEq/L
	Osmolarity
	• 0.9%: 308 mOsm/L
	• 3%: 1026 mOsm/L
	• 7.5%: 2565 mOsm/L
	• 23.4%: 8008 mOsm/L

constriction of cerebral vessels, thereby reducing intracerebral blood volume and ICP. Most studies suggest that in order for hyperosmolar therapy to be of any benefit, the blood-brain barrier must be intact. It is thought that in areas of injury where the blood-brain barrier has been compromised, the osmotic agent may pass through the membrane and equilibrate between blood and the interstitial fluid. Thus, these agents may remove water only from the normal healthy brain tissue and have minimal effect on the damaged area.[1] This may allow enough change in cerebral volume to accommodate the pressure increase produced by damaged tissue, but may be limited by stresses that the healthy tissue can tolerate.

CEREBRAL EDEMA

Cerebral edema is defined as an abnormal amount of fluid within the brain parenchyma resulting in a volumetric increase of the tissue,[9] and is generally classified into three major types: (1) cytotoxic, (2) vasogenic, and (3) interstitial. Cytotoxic edema results from failure of the ATP-dependent transport of sodium and calcium ions across the cell membrane leading to swelling of the neurons, glia, and endothelial cells.[3] Donkin and Vink[10] describe cytotoxic edema as a shift of water within the skull, with the water shifting from the extracellular to the intracellular compartment. Cytotoxic edema is most often seen in ischemic stroke and severe TBIs, affects gray and white matter, and is resistant to standard medical treatment including osmotic agents.[3,9,11–13] Vasogenic edema, however, occurs when water shifts from the vasculature to the extracellular space in response to an osmotic gradient created by vascular components permeating into the brain parenchyma.[10] Vasogenic edema is commonly seen in tissue hypoxia, intracerebral hemorrhages, water intoxication, trauma, tumor, cerebral abscesses, and other inflammatory conditions. Unlike cytotoxic edema, vasogenic edema is usually responsive to hyperosmolar and steroid therapy.[3] Lastly, interstitial edema is caused by increased pressure of the CSF leading to increased transependymal flow of CSF. This ultimately results in edema of the brain tissue lining the ventricles. Although not responsive to steroids, evidence suggests this particular edema may be responsive to osmotic therapy.[3] Of note, neurologic insults and injuries usually involve a combination of the different types of cerebral edema, although one type may predominate depending on the nature and duration of the injury. Forsyth and colleagues[14] note that cytotoxic edema usually occurs over minutes to hours after an injury, whereas vasogenic occurs hours to days postinjury. Given the variable responses of each type of edema, it is important to note the type of cerebral edema present when considering therapy. It is also important to note that cerebral edema may be localized or global.

HISTORICAL BACKGROUND

The concept of osmotherapy for central nervous disorders dates back almost a century. In 1919 two research fellows, Weed and McKibben,[15] discovered intravenous injections of concentrated 30% sodium chloride solution into anesthetized cats caused the normal convexity of the brain to shrink approximately 3 to 4 mm below the inner table of the skull. Later that year, Haden[16] reported on two cases using hypertonic glucose solutions for the treatment of cerebral edema in the setting of meningitis. A few years later, in 1927, intravenous administration of concentrated urea was introduced to the clinical setting by Fremont-Smith and Forbes,[17] although urea would not be regularly used until the 1950s.[18] Meanwhile other osmotic agents continued to be evaluated. In 1938, Hughes and colleagues[19] reported on the use of quad-concentrated plasma proteins as a possible treatment of increased ICP. By 1962, Wise and Chater[20] found that mannitol had the benefits of longer ICP control, less "rebound overshoot" than urea, stability in solution, less risk of toxicity, and low cost. After these discoveries mannitol remained the recommended osmotic therapy agent of choice for decades. It was not until 1985 that Todd and colleagues[21] again demonstrated the cerebral effects of hypertonic saline on ICP and cerebral blood flow in experiments with rabbits. With the addition of hypertonic saline for treatment of elevated ICP, the literature has now focused on determining which of these two agents is more appropriate and effective.

PHARMACOLOGIC PROPERTIES
Mannitol

Mannitol is a freely filtered nonmetabolized sugar alcohol that decreases the reabsorption of water and sodium across the renal tubules, creating a diuretic effect. Mannitol has been considered a cornerstone in the medical management of cerebral edema for the past several decades. The Brain Trauma Foundation and the European Brain Injury Consortium have identified level II and III evidence to support the use of mannitol in patients with elevated ICPs after a TBI. Data suggest that mannitol works in a biphasic fashion to reduce ICP. First, it decreases the viscosity of the blood. This allows the red blood cell to pass more easily through the vasculature independent of hematocrit, improving regional cerebral microvascular flow and oxygenation.[22,23] Although the effects of mannitol during this phase are immediate, evidence suggests that this effect peaks within approximately 30 minutes and diminishes about 4 to 6 hours after administration.[22–25] Mannitol also increases intravascular volume because of increased plasma osmolality pulling volume from the tissue intravascularly. This may have the added benefit of increasing cardiac output if preload is lacking, but does put the patient at risk for intravascular volume overload if they have poor cardiac or renal function. Assuming autoregulation is intact, there is a compensatory cerebral vasoconstriction that occurs in response to reduced viscosity and intravascular volume expansion. If autoregulation is impaired, reduction in ICP may be modest or absent.[22,23] The second phase of ICP reduction transpires as mannitol shifts fluid from the extracellular space into the intravascular compartment via the osmotic gradient. It is thought that for the mannitol to successfully extract water, an intact blood-brain barrier must be present. However, there is still debate around whether the volume is removed from injured or uninjured tissue. It seems that both injured and uninjured tissues may contribute to the volume of water eliminated, particularly in TBI. However most data suggest uninjured brain seems to be the main source of water extraction, especially with repeat dosing in ischemic stroke.[22] Ziai and colleagues[3] report other properties of mannitol include reduction in systemic vascular resistance (and hence afterload), combined with transiently increased preload and a mild positive inotropic effect resulting in improved cardiac output and oxygen delivery. Mannitol also acts as a free radical scavenger with potential cytoprotection by reducing the harmful effects of free radicals during ischemia-reperfusion injury.[22,23] However, intravascular volume is reduced following its diuretic effect because the kidneys work to remove excess intravascular volume, therefore fluid status should be assessed to avoid hypovolemia resulting in hypotension and secondary ischemic injury or elevation of ICP caused by reflex vasodilation of cerebral arterioles. Mannitol is generally dosed 0.25 g/kg to 1 g/kg. However, depending on dose and patient's total body water content, serum sodium may decrease 9 mEq/L to 13 mEq/L and should be monitored to prevent dramatic shifts in sodium.[22] The reduction of serum sodium occurs because its resorption across the renal tubule is inhibited by mannitol. The excretion of mannitol is essentially dependent on glomerular filtration rate (GFR). Presuming a patient has normal GFR and total body water, plasma mannitol concentration should be minimal after 4 hours, and may be readministered at that time as clinically indicated.[22]

Hypertonic Saline

Hypertonic saline is a less potent diuretic compared with mannitol. Unlike mannitol, it expands the intravascular volume, increases blood pressure, and theoretically increases cerebral blood flow in a more sustained fashion. It is hypothesized that hypertonic saline produces a diuretic effect by stimulating the release of atrial natriuretic peptide versus direct osmotic diuresis, thus explaining its ability to augment intravascular volume and cardiac performance.[3] Consequently, hypovolemia and hypotension are not common. Improved cerebral blood flow and oxygen delivery are believed to occur via dehydration of cerebrovascular endothelial cells, resulting in increased vessel diameter and improving deformability of red blood cells.[3] As Fink[8] points out, the osmotic load from hypertonic saline increases blood volume and MAP while at the same time decreasing ICP. Similar to mannitol, hypertonic saline has also been shown to produce a biphasic reduction in ICP; initially by creating rheologic changes followed by osmotic shifts across the blood-brain barrier. Theoretically, hypertonic saline is less permeable than mannitol when crossing the blood-brain barrier because of its higher reflection coefficient, thus the potential for water to follow the solute into the brain worsening cerebral edema is reduced.[22] Given there is no universally agreed on concentration for administering hypertonic saline, comparison among studies is difficult. The literature contains reference to hypertonic saline concentrations ranging from 3% to 23.5% sodium chloride. Additionally, the question of whether hypertonic saline is best administered on a bolus schedule versus a continuous infusion (or even mixed regimen) is unclear. Mortazavi and colleagues[26] performed a recent meta-analysis on the use of hypertonic saline for elevated ICP in patients with a variety of neurologic injuries and insults. The analysis included a total of 36 studies, which were a combination of retrospective, prospective observational, prospective nonrandomized, and randomized controlled trials. In the analysis, hypertonic saline was administered as a continuous infusion in 11 of the included studies. Six of these studies titrated the hypertonic saline infusions based on a goal serum sodium range,[27–32] whereas four titrated the infusions to a target ICP level.[33–36] The remaining study used a continuous infusion over 3 days in postoperative neurosurgery patients.[37] Multiple studies in the meta-analysis suggest that hypertonic saline administered as a continuous infusion is an effective method of reducing ICP. However, the retrospective study performed by Qureshi and colleagues[29] found no significant difference in ICP between patients with TBI who received hypertonic saline and those who received normal saline. In fact, the in-hospital mortality rate was higher in those who received hypertonic saline. Of note, worse outcome after hypertonic saline was not noted in any bolus study. Two out of three randomized controlled trials in the analysis support the use of hypertonic saline as a continuous infusion, compared with six of seven randomized controlled trials in which hypertonic boluses were used. Although there is significantly more data on hypertonic saline administration in bolus form versus continuous infusion, the available data do suggest that both routes are effective in reducing ICP depending on the patient subset.

CLINICAL APPLICATIONS IN VARIOUS PATIENT SUBSETS
Traumatic Brain Injuries

Most of the research on hyperosmolar therapy in neurologic injury has been performed in the TBI population. However, even in this particular population the evidence available ranges from class II to III. According to Ropper,[1] in patients with TBI, a single dose of mannitol reduces ICP within 10 to 15 minutes, with a maximal effect of decreasing the initial pressure by approximately 50% in 20 to 60 minutes. Despite the fact mannitol improves MAP, CPP, and CBF while lowering ICP initially, as Hinson and colleagues[22] point out, mannitol becomes less effective with repeat dosing and has numerous adverse effects. Given these side effects, more recent literature cites hypertonic saline as an effective alternative to mannitol in the TBI population. The literature initially reports findings in which continuous infusions of hypertonic saline were investigated. Qureshi and colleagues[28] found that a continuous infusion of 3% saline exerted a beneficial effect on ICP and improved lateral displacement of brain caused by edema in patients with head injuries. However, like mannitol, bolus dosing of hypertonic saline has shown more promise in patients with TBI than continuous infusions because they allow more time for the re-establishment of a new osmotic set point, such that the intracellular and extracellular compartments are able to re-equilibrate.[22] No further water extraction can occur once the re-equilibration occurs. Hinson and colleagues[22] also cite several case series that have shown the effectiveness of boluses of hypertonic saline for the reduction of ICP in TBI, as an alternative and as an adjuvant to mannitol.

Ischemic Stroke

Unlike TBI, the utility of hyperosmolar agents in ischemic stroke is still highly debated. To date, there has not been a randomized controlled trial addressing the use of mannitol in the ischemic stroke population. In fact, some of the literature even points to the possibility of negative effects from mannitol.[38] Despite the absence of definitive evidence in humans, mannitol rescue therapy for malignant cerebral edema is the most common clinical practice. The American Stroke Association guidelines recommend the use of mannitol when treating elevated ICP and cerebral edema in the stroke population until more definitive therapy, such as decompressive craniectomy, can be performed.[22] The utility of using hypertonic saline in patients with ischemic stroke is just as unclear. A study in eight patients with ischemic stroke found that bolus infusions of hypertonic saline consistently led to an almost immediate and substantial decrease in an acutely raised ICP and to a marked rise in CPP.[39] Additionally, in all of these patients previous treatment with mannitol had not been effective. However, there are concerns for using hyperosmolar therapy in the ischemic stroke population.

The first concern surrounds the lack of intact blood-brain barrier in this particular patient population. Theoretically, osmotic agents may leak across the compromised membrane leading to increased water in the injured area as it follows the solute. Although this phenomenon has been reported in animals, it has not been conclusively demonstrated in humans. The second concern is that mannitol may preferentially reduce the water content of the uninjured hemisphere, which could worsen midline shifts if this occurs. To address these concerns, Manno and colleagues[40] studied a group of patients with large middle cerebral artery infarctions who had received mannitol in the setting of cerebral edema and elevated ICP. They concluded that a single large dose of mannitol (1.5 g/kg of body weight) did not worsen midline shift or precipitate neurologic decline within the first hour after administration. Although the literature suggests bolus dosing of mannitol and hypertonic saline can reduce ICPs in ischemic stroke, long-term outcomes in these studies were not addressed. Therefore, until further research is performed the precise role of these two agents in the ischemic stroke population remains to be seen.

Subarachnoid Hemorrhage

Evidence has shown that mannitol and hypertonic saline significantly lower ICP in animal models with subarachnoid hemorrhage, but little research comparing the two agents has been performed in humans. This is likely because of the concern that diuresis caused by the administration of mannitol may induce cerebral vasospasm. In a Norwegian study that compared 7.2% hypertonic saline with a placebo of normal saline in stable patients with subarachnoid hemorrhage, hypertonic saline was found to decrease ICP 3 mm Hg on average compared with 0.3 mm Hg in the placebo group.[41] It seems that the authors correctly hypothesized that hypertonic saline would be more successful in lowering ICP given a relatively intact blood-brain barrier. A study by Tseng and colleagues[42] concluded that infusions of 23.5% hypertonic saline not only reduced ICP in poor grade subarachnoid patients, but also increased cerebral blood flow as evidenced by continuous transcranial Doppler and xenon-enhanced computed tomography scans.

Intracerebral Hemorrhage

Evidence for the use of hyperosmotic agents in patients with intracerebral hemorrhage is lacking. In 2005 Misra and colleagues[43] published a study that included 128 patients with spontaneous intracerebral hemorrhage who were randomized to low-dose mannitol versus placebo. Results concluded that patients who received scheduled, low-dose mannitol (100 mL of 20% dosed every 4 hours) did not improve outcomes or change cerebral blood flow. Other than a case report, no clinical trials in which human patients with intracerebral hemorrhage received hypertonic saline alone could be identified. To date, published studies include patients who received a combination of mannitol and hypertonic saline, or hypertonic saline with hetastarch, or patients who had an intracerebral hemorrhage as part of a larger cohort of varying neurologic injuries.

Transtentorial Herniation

In 2000 Qureshi and colleagues[44] published a study that found hyperventilation in combination with mannitol reversed transtentorial herniation in a cohort of 28 patients with varying underlying neurologic injuries. As previously discussed in the 2012 meta-analysis by Mortazavi and colleagues[26], hypertonic saline might be more effective than mannitol in reducing episodes of increased ICP, but the state of the literature is limited by small sample sizes and inconsistent study methods. A retrospective cohort study by Koenig and colleagues[45] evaluated the role of 23.4% saline in the management of 76 transtentorial herniation events in 68 patients with subarachnoid hemorrhages, intracerebral hemorrhages, tumors, subdural hematomas, epidural hematomas, and meningitis. In addition to hypertonic saline other treatment measures included hyperventilation, mannitol, propofol, pentobarbital, ventriculostomy drainage, and decompressive craniotomy. Results showed a reversal of transtentorial herniation in 75% of the 76 events. Ultimately 22 of the patients survived until discharge with varying degrees of disabilities.

MONITORING

Given that hyperosmolar agents are typically used in clinical scenarios that include elevated ICP and impending herniation, it is recommended to have an ICP monitor in place to aid in titration of hyperosmolar therapy and trending of ICP. Based on the available data, the authors recommend that regardless of which hyperosmolar agent is selected, fluid balance should be closely monitored because mannitol may cause significant diuresis leading to hypovolemia, whereas hypertonic saline expands intravascular volume and can lead to fluid overload. Serial serum sodium and plasma osmolality are frequently obtained after the administration of either hypertonic saline or mannitol. Target serum sodium and osmolality values are debated, but clinicians typically aim for serum sodium concentrations of 150 mEq/L to 160 mEq/L and plasma osmolality between 300 mOsm and 320 mOsm. Regardless of the baseline sodium concentration, an infusion of 1 mL/kg of 3% saline generally raises the serum sodium by approximately 1 mEq/L.[22] Hinson and colleagues[22] claim that despite its frequent clinical use, serum osmolality is a poor surrogate for serum mannitol concentrations. Instead, they advocate the use of osmolar gap as a way of monitoring mannitol concentrations to avoid complications. The osmolar gap is obtained by finding the difference between the measured osmolality by laboratory sample from the calculated osmolarity. Although osmolar gap is calculated in a variety of ways, Diringer and Zazulia[46] report that using $1.86(Na^+ + K^+) + (blood, urea, nitrogen/2.8) + (glucose/18) + 10$ as the calculation for osmolarity provided the best correlation to measured mannitol levels. Evidence suggests that an osmolar gap less than 55 mmol/kg of H_2O is needed to prevent renal failure.[22]

COMPLICATIONS
Renal Failure

Renal failure is one of the most common complications of mannitol. Hinson and colleagues[22] point out that mannitol can cause nephrotoxicity by several mechanisms including dose-dependent vasoconstriction of the renal artery and intravascular volume depletion from osmotic diuresis. Dorman and colleagues[47] observed that the mean total dose of mannitol required to prompt acute renal failure in healthy kidneys was 626 ± 270 g over 2 to 5 days. Although reports of renal failure associated with the use of hypertonic saline are limited, close monitoring of renal function is recommended. Although the use of mannitol in patients who have a history of renal failure is not advised, if used the smallest effective dose possible should be administered (consider 0.5 g/kg). In patients with GFR less than 50 mL/min, hemodialysis decreases the half-life of mannitol to 6 hours versus 5 or more days.[22]

Osmotic Demyelinating Syndrome

Osmotic demyelinating syndrome or central pontine myelinolysis (CPM) may occur if sodium levels are rapidly increased. This syndrome causes destruction of the myelin sheath and can lead to serious long-term disability. Patients who are hyponatremic at baseline are at a higher risk for developing CPM. To date, there are no case reports of CPM occurring after the administration of hypertonic saline for the treatment of intracranial hypertension.[22]

Rebound Phenomenon

A patient's ICP may initially rise after receiving hyperosmolar therapy.[22,39] Known as the "rebound phenomenon," it is more commonly seen after mannitol administration. At one point, it was thought that this rebound effect occurred secondary to the osmotic agent permeating into injured tissue, pulling water with it. However, Hinson and colleagues[22] suggest that the temporary increase in ICP is more likely caused by an osmotic compensation within the central nervous system that allows for increased intracellular concentrations of electrolytes. Repeated administration of osmotic agents, especially without allowing time for the medication to clear before the next dose, may promote the rebound phenomenon.[22]

Acid/Base Imbalances and Other Complications

Not only does hypertonic saline inhibit the resorption of bicarbonate from the proximal renal tubules, it may also produce hyperchloremic metabolic acidosis secondary to the large load of chloride that is delivered with each dose.[22] Other adverse effects that may occur can include but are not limited to other electrolyte imbalances and seizures. Mannitol may cause a hypokalemic and hypochloremic alkalosis secondary to volume contraction and diuresis leading to hypotension. In contrast, hypertonic saline may lead to congestive heart failure secondary to increased intravascular volume.

SUMMARY

As Kamel and colleagues[48] point out, several studies have suggested that hypertonic saline may be superior to mannitol in reducing ICP, but the impact of these studies on clinical practice has been limited. This is partly because of the different formulations of mannitol and hypertonic saline used and partly because of the small sample size of these studies. The meta-analysis by Mortazavi and colleagues[26] found that in 9 of the 12 studies that compared hypertonic saline with mannitol, including seven randomized controlled trials, data suggest that hypertonic saline proved superior to mannitol in decreasing ICPs. They found that there was a greater reduction in ICP in the minutes to hours following administration. A longer duration of effect was found in two studies, and one randomized controlled trial found that the number of episodes of elevated ICP were lower in patients who received hypertonic saline than those who received mannitol. However, mortality rates and overall neurologic outcomes were not consistent among the trials. Given there is no level I evidence that compares hypertonic saline with mannitol, more rigorous clinical data are needed.

REFERENCES

1. Ropper AH. Hyperosmolar therapy for raised intracranial pressure. N Engl J Med 2012;367(8):746–52.
2. Faul M, Xu L, Wald MM, et al. Traumatic brain injury in the United States: emergency department visits, hospitalizations and deaths 2002–2006. Atlanta (GA): Centers for Disease Control and Prevention, National Center for Injury Prevention and Control; 2010.
3. Ziai WC, Toung TJ, Bhardwaj A. Hypertonic saline: first-line therapy for cerebral edema. J Neurol Sci 2007;261:157–66.

4. Mokri B. The Monro-Kellie hypothesis applications in CSF volume depletion. Neurology 2001;56:1746–8.
5. Lundberg N. The saga of the Monro-Kellie doctrine. In: Ishii S, Nagai H, Brock M, editors. Intracranial pressure V: proceedings of the fifth International Symposium on Intracranial Pressure, held at Tokyo, Japan, May 30-June 3, 1982. Berlin: Springer Science & Business Media; 1983. p. 68–76.
6. Monro A. Observations on the structure and function of the nervous system: illustrated with tables. Edinburgh (United Kingdom): Creech and Johnson; 1783.
7. Kellie G. An account of the appearances observed in the dissection of two of three individuals presumed to have perished in the storm of the 3rd, and whose bodies were discovered in the vicinity of Leith on the morning of the 4th November 1821 with some reflections on the pathology of the brain. Med Chir Trans 1824;1:84–169.
8. Fink ME. Osmotherapy for intracranial hypertension: mannitol versus hypertonic saline. Continuum Lifelong Learn Neurol 2012;18(3):640–54.
9. Klatzo I. Pathophysiological aspects of brain edema. Acta Neuropathol 1987; 72(3):236.
10. Donkin JJ, Vink R. Mechanisms of cerebral edema in traumatic brain injury: therapeutic developments. Curr Opin Neurol 2010;23:293–9.
11. Caplan LR. Basic pathology, anatomy, and pathophysiology of stroke. In: Caplan's stroke: a clinical approach. 4th edition. Philadelphia: Saunders Elsevier; 2009. p. 22.
12. Deb P, Sharma S, Hassan KM. Pathophysiologic mechanisms of acute ischemic stroke: an overview with emphasis on therapeutic significance beyond thrombolysis. Pathophysiology 2010;17(3):197.
13. Simard JM, Kent TA, Chen M, et al. Brain oedema in focal ischaemia: molecular pathophysiology and theoretical implications. Lancet Neurol 2007;6(3):258.
14. Forsyth LL, Liu-DeRyke X, Parker D Jr, et al. Role of hypertonic saline for the management of intracranial hypertension after stroke and traumatic brain injury. Pharmacotherapy 2008;28:469–84.
15. Weed LH, McKibben PS. Experimental alteration of brain bulk. Am J Physiol 1919; 48:531–55.
16. Haden R. Therapeutic application of the alteration of brain volume by the intravenous injection of glucose. JAMA 1919;73(13):983–4.
17. Fremont-Smith F, Forbes HS. Intraocular and intracranial pressure: an experimental study. Arch Neur Psych 1927;18:555–64.
18. Rosomoff HL. Distribution of intracranial contents after hypertonic urea. J Neurosurg 1962;19(10):859–64.
19. Hughes J, Mudd S, Strecker EA. Reduction of increased intracranial pressure by concentrated solutions of human lyophile serum. Arch Neur Psych 1938;39(6): 1277–87.
20. Wise BL, Chater N. The value of hypertonic mannitol solution in decreasing brain mass and lowering cerebro-spinal-fluid pressure. J Neurosurg 1962;19:1038–43.
21. Todd MM, Tommasino C, Moore S. Cerebral effects of isovolemic hemodilution with hypertonic saline solution. J Neurosurg 1985;63:944–8.
22. Hinson HE, Stein D, Sheth KN. Hypertonic saline and mannitol therapy in critical care neurology. J Intensive Care Med 2010;28(1):3–11.
23. Shawkat H, Westwood M, Mortimer A. Mannitol: a review of its clinical uses. continuing education in anaesthesia. Crit Care Pain 2012;12(2):82–5.
24. Dennis LJ, Mayer SA. Diagnosis and management of increased intracranial pressure. Neurol India 2001;49(S1):S37.

25. Jafar JJ, Johns LM, Mullan SF. The effect of mannitol on cerebral blood flow. J Neurosurg 1986;64(5):754.
26. Mortazavi M, Romeo AK, Deep A, et al. Hypertonic saline for treating raised intra-cranial pressure: literature review with meta-analysis. J Neurosurg 2012;116: 210–21.
27. Larive LL, Rhoney DH, Parker D Jr, et al. Introducing hypertonic saline for cere-bral edema: an academic center experience. Neurocrit Care 2004;1:435–40.
28. Qureshi AI, Suarez JI, Bhardwaj A, et al. Use of hypertonic (3%) saline/acetate infusion in the treatment of cerebral edema: effect on intracranial pressure and lateral displacement of the brain. Crit Care Med 1998;26:440–6.
29. Qureshi AI, Suarez JI, Castro A, et al. Use of hypertonic saline/acetate infusion in treatment of cerebral edema in patients with head trauma: experience at a single center. J Trauma 1999;47:659–65.
30. Rockswold GL, Solid CA, Paredes-Andrade E, et al. Hypertonic saline and its ef-fect on intracranial pressure, cerebral perfusion pressure, and brain tissue oxy-gen. Neurosurgery 2009;65:1035–42.
31. Simma B, Burger R, Falk M, et al. A prospective, randomized, and controlled study of fluid management in children with severe head injury: lactated Ringer's solution versus hypertonic saline. Crit Care Med 1998;26:1265–70.
32. Yildizdas D, Altunbasak S, Celik U, et al. Hypertonic saline treatment in children with cerebral edema. Indian Pediatr 2016;43:771–9.
33. Härtl R, Ghajar J, Hochleuthner H, et al. Hypertonic/hyperoncotic saline reliably reduces ICP in severely head injured patients with intracranial hypertension. Acta Neurochir 1997;S70:126–9.
34. Harutjunyan L, Holz C, Rieger A, et al. Efficiency of 7.2% hypertonic saline hy-droxyethyl starch 200/0.5 versus mannitol 15% in the treatment of increased intra-cranial pressure in neurosurgical patients: a randomized clinical trial. Crit Care 2005;9:R530–40.
35. Khanna S, Davis D, Peterson B, et al. Use of hypertonic saline in the treatment of severe refractory posttraumatic intracranial hypertension in pediatric traumatic brain injury. Crit Care Med 2000;28:1144–51.
36. Peterson B, Khanna S, Fisher B, et al. Prolonged hypernatremia controls elevated intracranial pressure in head-injured pediatric patients. Crit Care Med 2000;28: 1136–43.
37. De Vivo P, Del Gaudio A, Ciritella P, et al. Hypertonic saline solution: a safe alter-native to mannitol 18% in neurosurgery. Minerva Anestesiol 2001;67:603–11.
38. Bereczki D, Mihálka L, Szatmári S, et al. Mannitol use in acute stroke case fatality at 30 days and 1 year. Stroke 2003;4(7):1730–5.
39. Schwartz S, Georgiadis D, Aschoff A, et al. Effects of hypertonic (10%) saline in patients with raised intracranial pressure after stroke. Stroke 2002;33:136–40.
40. Manno EM, Adams RE, Derdeyn CP, et al. The effects of mannitol on cerebral edema after large hemispheric cerebral infarct. Neurology 1999;52(3):583–7.
41. Bentsen G, Breivik H, Lundar T, et al. Hypertonic saline (7.2%) in 6% hydroxyethyl starch reduces intracranial pressure and improves hemodynamics in a place-controlled study involving stable patients with subarachnoid hemorrhage. Crit Care Med 2006;34(12):2912–7.
42. Tseng MY, Al-Rawi PG, Czosnyka M, et al. Enhancement of cerebral blood flow using systemic hypertonic saline therapy improves outcome in patients with poor-grade spontaneous subarachnoid hemorrhage. J Neurosurg 2007;107(2): 274–82.

43. Misra UK, Kalita J, Ranjan P, et al. Mannitol in intracerebral hemorrhage: a randomized controlled study. J Neurol Sci 2005;234(1–2):41–5.
44. Qureshi AI, Geocadin RG, Suarez JI, et al. Long-term outcomes after medical reversal of transtentorial herniation in patients with supratentorial mass lesions. Crit Care Med 2000;28(5):1556–64.
45. Koenig MA, Bryan M, Lewis JL, et al. Reversal of transtentorial herniation with hypertonic saline. Neurology 2008;70:1023–9.
46. Diringer MN, Zazulia AR. Osmotic therapy: fact and fiction. Neurocrit Care 2004; 1(2):219–33.
47. Dorman HR, Sondheimer JH, Cadnapaphornchai P. Mannitol induced acute renal failure. Medicine 1990;69(3):153–9.
48. Kamel H, Navi BB, Nakagawa K, et al. Hypertonic saline versus mannitol for the treatment of elevated intracranial pressure: a meta-analysis of randomized clinical trials. Crit Care Med 2011;39:554–9.

Does Evidence Drive Fluid Volume Restriction in Chronic Heart Failure?

Robin K. Miller, MSN, ACNP-BC, CHFN[a,b,*],
Nathaniel Thornton, MN, AGACNP-BC[c]

KEYWORDS

- Heart failure • Fluid restriction • Thirst • Adherence

KEY POINTS

- Fluid restriction is an aspect of heart failure education and management.
- There is no expert consensus on the degree of fluid restriction that is recommended.
- Congestion leads to an increase in symptom burden and disease progression and is target of heart failure therapies.
- Thirst is a common complaint in heart failure patients and can decrease adherence to fluid restriction.

With a changing and aging population, chronic heart failure (HF) remains a challenge to treat with acute decompensations resulting in costly hospital admissions.[1] This complex clinical syndrome is associated with a high degree of mortality and morbidity. Treatment approaches include both pharmacologic and nonpharmacologic strategies. Fluid restriction in chronic HF patients has been a core tenet of education and management plans, but the question remains whether the evidence supports the practice.

Funding Sources: None.
Conflict of Interest: None.
[a] Heart Failure and Transplant, Knight Cardiovascular Institute, Oregon Health and Science University, 3181 SW Sam Jackson Park Road, Portland, OR 97239, USA; [b] Adult-Gerontology Acute Care Nurse Practitioner Program, Oregon Health and Science University, 3181 SW Sam Jackson Park Road, Portland, OR 97239, USA; [c] School of Nursing, Oregon Health and Science University, 3181 SW Sam Jackson Park Road, Portland, OR 97239, USA
* Corresponding author. Oregon Health and Science University, 3181 SW Sam Jackson Park Road, Portland, OR 97239.
E-mail address: millero@ohsu.edu

PATHOPHYSIOLOGY OF HEART FAILURE

HF is characterized by structural and functional impairments in ventricular filling and emptying, leading to a complex set of physical manifestations such as dyspnea, fatigue, and edema.[1,2] The primary driver of these symptoms, and the attributable morbidity and mortality, is thought to be related to congestion. Congestion is an end result of a complex pathophysiologic cascade characterized by alterations in cardiac output. This low cardiac output state impairs renal perfusion, leading to activation of the sympathetic nervous and renin-angiotensin-aldosterone systems with the end result being increased renal sodium and water retention and increased circulating blood volume.[3,4] Chronic activation of these pathways leads to ventricular remodeling and progressive cardiac impairment,[5] which leads to increased sodium and water retention and, ultimately, congestion.

Beta-blockers, mineralocorticoid receptor antagonists, and angiotensin-converting-enzyme inhibitors/angiotensin II receptor blockers constitute the core pharmacologic strategies used in chronic HF.[2] These targeted pharmacologic management strategies of HF are focused on blocking the maladaptive neurohormonal processes inherent in HF. Volume control is essential to preventing congestion, which is accomplished through the use of diuretics, self-care strategies that incorporate sodium and fluid restriction, and daily weight measurements.[6,7] Nonpharmacologic approaches to volume management rely heavily on a degree of patient self-care, which is influenced by physical, psychological, environmental, and social factors.[8] Thirst related to the maladaptive disease progression and management strategies is a common complaint in those with late-stage HF.[1] Together, these pharmacologic and non-pharmacologic management strategies aim to prevent both progression and acute decompensation episodes of chronic HF.[2]

FLUID RESTRICTION: CURRENT STATE OF EVIDENCE

Fluid restriction is recommended in current HF management guidelines, but the science behind the recommendation has not been robust. There is presumption that non-adherence to a sodium and fluid–restricted diet can be a contributing factor to decompensation.[2] Based on this supposition, coupled with clinical opinion and experience, fluid restriction remains part of current HF guidelines.

GUIDELINES

Current guidelines for fluid restriction in chronic HF are summarized in **Table 1**. The American Heart Association (AHA), European Society of Cardiology (ESC), and Heart Failure Society of America (HFSA) all have published guidelines for the management of chronic HF, including dietary considerations.[1,2,9] Fluid restriction, although included in some iteration of all published guidelines, is supported by expert opinion as opposed to concrete clinical evidence from randomized controlled trials (RCTs).[10]

There is currently no consensus on a specific level of fluid restriction for all patients with HF. In those patients with congestive symptoms, there is agreement that fluid restriction is warranted, although the degree of fluid restriction differs among the groups.[1,2,9] Both the AHA and the ESC recommend fluid restrictions in those with stage D or severe HF.[1,2] Hyponatremia is a concerning feature of HF and is associated with increased mortality[11,12]; both the AHA and the ESC guidelines prompt fluid restriction in scenarios of hyponatremia and end-stage HF.[1,2] The HFSA[9] guidelines stipulate that fluid restriction should be considered when congestion persists despite high-dose diuretics and sodium restriction. Only the

Table 1
American Heart Association, European Society of Cardiology, Heart Failure Society of America guidelines for fluid restriction

Guidelines	American Heart Association[2]	European Society of Cardiology[1]	Heart Failure Society of America[9]
	Fluid restriction up to 1.5 to 2 L/d is reasonable for patients in stage D ± hyponatremia, to reduce congestive symptoms	Fluid restriction up to 1.5 to 2 L/d is reasonable for patients in stage D ± hyponatremia, to reduce congestive symptoms Weight-based fluid restriction (30 mL/kg, 35 mL/kg if body weight >85 kg) may cause less thirst	Fluid restriction up to 1.5 to 2 L/d is reasonable for patients in stage D ± hyponatremia, to reduce congestive symptoms

Data from Refs.[1,2,9]

ESC guidelines address thirst,[1] a common complaint in HF patients, using a weight-based fluid restriction recommendation.

RANDOMIZED CONTROLLED TRIALS

Despite the lack of concrete evidence and RCTs, fluid restriction is commonly prescribed by HF providers as part of a disease management program.[13–15] To date, there are only 7 available RCTs, each with conflicting and differing degrees of restrictions and benefits derived from fluid restriction.[5,16–21] Of the 7 studies available, all the sample sizes were small, ranging from 46 to 75 in all but one, sample size of 97, of the available trials.[5,16–20] Only 2 studies looked at fluid restriction in isolation,[18,20] whereas the others included fluid restriction in conjunction with sodium restriction or other dietary modifications.[5,16,17,19,21] Variations in prescribed fluid restrictions also make comparison challenging.

Four studies reported beneficial effects of fluid restriction in those with HF. The most commonly reported benefit was increased quality of life (QoL).[5,16,19] One study only looked at fluid restriction comparisons of 1 L versus 2 L.[16] Two others examined the effect of a 1.5-L/d fluid restriction in conjunction with either a sodium restriction[19] or a sodium restriction with a nutritional education.[5] Paterna and colleagues[21] examined the impact of fluid restriction, diuretic dose, and sodium restriction in those with recently compensated HF. They found that the group with the more stringent fluid and sodium restriction (1 L and 120 mmol/d, respectively), in addition to high-dose diuretics (500 mg furosemide), had lower rates of hospital readmission.[21]

Of the remaining 3 studies, there were no demonstrated benefits of fluid restriction.[17,18,20] Both Aliti and colleagues[17] and Travers and colleagues[20] looked at decompensated HF patients, and neither study revealed changes in clinical stability in the fluid-restricted group. In addition, neither of these studies examined fluid restriction and clinical stability in compensated chronic HF patients. Another study examined chronic HF patients with a restricted fluid diet (1.5 L) versus liberal fluid intake, and the former was associated with increased perception of thirst and worse adherence in fluid-restricted patients.[18] There is some evidence that, in the short term, a strict fluid restriction can assist with decongestion of those in decompensated HF—however, there were no sustained long-term benefits demonstrated.[20,22]

AREAS OF CONSIDERATION

Fluid restriction, although long considered a standard of HF management, is not universally supported in the literature. Even in those RCTs that found benefit related to fluid restriction, there were no overwhelming or significant changes in rates of hospitalization and mortality.[22,23] QoL was the most commonly cited benefit in these groups.[5,16] For those living with HF, improvement in QoL is key to achieving success with treatment programs.[24] The morbidities associated with HF often impact adherence to both pharmacologic and nonpharmacologic treatment strategies. Self-care becomes an essential tenant of HF management. Thirst, sodium restriction, and hyponatremia are all competing aspects of HF management that may impact adherence to fluid restriction—all causes for nonadherence of self-care directed nonpharmacologic strategies.[8]

Thirst

The perception of thirst can be a distressing symptom for HF patients. The activation of neurohormonal pathways leads to stimulation of the thirst center in the hypothalamus.[17] The perception of thirst can be accentuated by xerostomia (dryness of the mouth) related to the use of diuretics.[25,26] Patients have reported that fluid restrictions are associated with intense thirst[16–18,27,28]; this association is independent of the degree of consumption. Adherence to prescribed fluid restrictions can be challenging, especially with the perception of intense thirst[26] and the common social, physical, and environmental factors that patients with fluid restriction are faced with.[8,24] Reilly and colleagues[29] found that adherence to fluid restriction was difficult, independent of education provided. The quality and intensity of thirst experienced by patients impacted adherence to prescribed therapies, especially dietary.[29] Adherence to the stringent dietary restrictions placed upon those with HF can be difficult to manage, even more so when associated with thirst.[30–32]

Sodium Restriction

Dietary sodium restrictions exist for the general healthy population and are incorporated in the current HF guidelines.[1,2,9] As seen with fluid restriction, there is no consensus on the degree of sodium restriction recommended, with wide variation in the levels of restriction in the available literature. Several of the RCTs detailed above incorporated sodium restriction and fluid restriction with mixed conclusions tied to the benefit of dietary restriction.[5,16,17,19,21] Other RCTs have been conducted solely examining sodium restriction in HF.[5,33–37] For those with sodium-restricted diets (800 mg/d to 1.5 mg/d), there were overall increases in activation of neurohormonal pathways leading to increased sodium and water retention.[33–37] One study demonstrated a decrease in patient-reported fatigue and edema with a sodium restriction (<2.4 g/d),[5] indicating a potential association with sodium restriction and congestion. There is insufficient evidence to suggest that a dietary sodium restriction alone is beneficial in chronic nondecompensated HF.[38] Coupling sodium and fluid restrictions with individualized education and support may increase adherence to HF management strategies.[15]

Hyponatremia

Hyponatremia is a common problem in patients with chronic HF and portends a poor prognosis.[39] The neurohormonal pathways activated in HF can cause worsening of serum sodium levels.[40] In those with chronic HF, hyponatremia is associated with increased hospitalizations, complications, and health care expenditures.[41,42]

Diuretics, used to pharmacologically manage volume status in chronic HF, are one of the most common causes of drug-induced hyponatremia.[43] Increased water retention from neurohormonal pathway activation is a contributing factor of hyponatremia, which leads to worsening congestion, further decreases in serum sodium levels, and baseline hyponatremia, all of which may limit provider use of diuretics.[40–43] To combat hyponatremia, free water restrictions may be implemented.[40] These restrictions, in conjunction with increased thirst, are associated with poor compliance, which can lead to further worsening hyponatremia associated with congestion.[29]

SUMMARY

HF is, by nature, predictably unpredictable, and the impact symptoms have on QoL cause considerable distress.[8] There is no conclusive evidence that fluid restriction alone is beneficial for compensated chronic HF patients, with very few RCTs available and conflicting reports of measureable benefits between the studies. Current guidelines still recommend some degree of fluid restriction for those with end-stage disease, hyponatremia, or symptoms of congestion, but these recommendations are based on expert opinion only, and there is no evidence to suggest that those with mild to moderate HF benefit from these measures.[13,14] It may instead be beneficial to continue to incorporate fluid restriction into larger clusters of self-care management strategies aimed at improving QoL and reducing symptom burden, as opposed to viewing fluid restriction in isolation.

REFERENCES

1. Ponikowski P, Voors AA, Anker SD, et al. 2016 ESC guidelines for the diagnosis and treatment of acute and chronic heart failure. Eur Heart J 2016;37(27): 2129–200.
2. Yancy CW, Jessup M, Bozkurt B, et al. 2013 ACCF/AHA guideline for the management of heart failure. Circulation 2013;128(16):e240–327.
3. Butler T. Dietary management of heart failure: room for improvement? Br J Nutr 2016;115(7):1202–17.
4. Houston BA, Kalathuya RJ, Kim DA, et al. Volume overload in heart failure: an evidence-based review of strategies for treatment and prevention. Mayo Clin Proc 2015;90(9):1247–61.
5. Colin-Ramirez E, Ezekowitz JA. Salt in the diet in patients with heart failure: what to recommend. Curr Opin Cardiol 2016;31(2):196–203.
6. D'Almeida KS, Rabelo-Silva ER, Souza GC, et al. Effect of fluid and dietary sodium restriction in the management of patients with heart failure and preserved ejection fraction: study protocol for a randomized controlled trial. Trials 2014; 15:347.
7. Stut W, Deighan C, Cleland JG, et al. Adherence to self-care in patients with heart failure in the HeartCycle study. Patient Prefer Adherence 2015;9:1195–206.
8. Strachen PH, Currie K, Harkness K, et al. Context matters in heart failure self-care: a qualitative systematic review. J Card Fail 2014;20(6):448–55.
9. Lindenfeld J, Albert NM, Boehmer JP, et al. HFSA 2010 comprehensive heart failure practice guidelines. J Card Fail 2010;16(6):e1–183.
10. Rami K. Aggressive salt and water restriction in acutely decompensated heart failure: is it worth its weight in salt? Expert Rev Cardiovasc Ther 2013;11(9): 1125–8.

11. Graudal NA, Hubeck-Graudal T, Jurgens G. Effects of low-sodium diet vs. high-sodium diet on blood pressure, renin, aldosterone, catecholamines, cholesterol, and triglyceride (Cochrane Review). Am J Hypertens 2012;25:1–25.
12. Sinkeler SJ, Damman K, van Veldhuisen DJ, et al. A re-appraisal of volume status and renal function impairment in chronic heart failure: combined effects of pre-renal failure and venous congestion on renal function. Heart Fail Rev 2012; 17(2):263–70.
13. Linhares JC, Aliti GB, Castro RA, et al. Prescribing and conducting non-pharmacological management of patients with decompensated heart failure admitted to a university hospital emergency. Rev Lat Am Enfermagem 2010;18: 1145–51.
14. Nieuwenhuis MM, Jaarsma T, van Veldhuisen DJ, et al. Long-term compliance with nonpharmacologic treatment of patients with heart failure. Am J Cardiol 2012;110(3):393–7.
15. Johansson P, van der Wal MHL, Stromberg A, et al. Fluid restriction in patients with heart failure: how should we think? Eur J Cardiovasc Nurs 2016;15(5):301–4.
16. Albert NM, Nutter B, Forney J, et al. A randomized controlled pilot study of outcomes of strict allowance of fluid therapy in hyponatremic heart failure (SALT-HF). J Card Fail 2013;19(1):1–9.
17. Aliti GB, Rabelo ER, Clausell N, et al. Aggressive fluid and sodium restriction in acute decompensated heart failure: a randomized clinical trial. JAMA Intern Med 2013;173(12):1058–64.
18. Holst M, Stromberg A, Lindholm M, et al. Liberal versus restricted fluid prescription in stabilized patients with chronic heart failure: result of a randomized crossover study of the effects on health-related quality of life. Scand Cardiovasc J 2008;42:316–22.
19. Philipson H, Ekman I, Forslund HB, et al. Salt and fluid restriction is effective in patients with chronic heart failure. Eur J Heart Fail 2013;15(11):1304–10.
20. Travers B, O'Loughlin C, Murphy NF, et al. Fluid restriction in the management of decompensated heart failure: no impact on time to clinical stability. J Card Fail 2007;13:128–32.
21. Paterna S, Parrinello G, Cannizzaro S, et al. Medium term effects of different dosage of diuretics, sodium, and fluid administration on neurohormonal and clinical outcome in patients with recently compensated heart failure. Am J Cardiol 2009;103:93–102.
22. de Veechis R, Baldi C, Cioppa C, et al. Effects of limiting fluid intake on clinical and laboratory outcomes in patients with heart failure: results of a meta-analysis of randomized control trials. Herz 2016;41(1):63–75.
23. Li Y, Fu B, Qian X. Liberal versus restricted fluid administration in heart failure patients. A systematic review and meta-analysis of randomized trials. Int Heart J 2015;56(2):192–5.
24. Dobre D, de Jongste MJL, Haaijer-Ruskamp FM, et al. The enigma of quality of life in patients with heart failure. Int J Cardiol 2008;125:407–9.
25. Allida SM, Inglis SC, Davidson PM, et al. Thirst in chronic heart failure: a review. J Clin Nurs 2015;24(7–8):916–26.
26. Waldréus N, Hahn RG, Lyngå P, et al. Changes in thirst intensity during optimization of heart failure medical therapy by nurses at the outpatient clinic. J Cardiovasc Nurs 2016;31(5):E17–24.
27. Shafazand M, Rosengren A, Lappas G, et al. Decreasing trends in the incidence of heart failure after acute myocardial infarction from 1993-2004: a study of

175,216 patients with a first acute myocardial infarction in Sweden. Eur J Heart Fail 2011;13:135–41.

28. Cereda E, Pedroli C, Lucchin L, et al. Fluid intake and nutritional risk in non-critically ill patients at hospital referral. Br J Nutr 2010;104:878–85.

29. Reilly CM, Higgins M, Smith A, et al. Isolating the benefits of fluid restriction in patients with heart failure: a pilot study. Eur J Cardiovasc Nurs 2015;14(6):494–505.

30. Welch JL, Thomas-Hawkins C. Psych-educational strategies to promote fluid adherence in adult hemodialysis patients. Int J Nurs Stud 2005;42:597–608.

31. Welch JL, Perkins SM, Evans JD, et al. Differences in perceptions by stage of fluid adherence. J Ren Nutr 2003;13:275–81.

32. Van der Wal MH, Jaarsma T, Moser DK, et al. Compliance in heart failure patients: the importance of knowledge and beliefs. Eur Heart J 2006;27:434–40.

33. Parrinello G, Torres D, Paterna S. Salt and water imbalance in chronic heart failure. Intern Emerg Med 2011;6(1):29–36.

34. Alvelos M, Ferreira A, Bettencourt P, et al. The effect of dietary sodium restriction on neurohormonal activity and renal dopaminergic response in patients with heart failure. Eur J Heart Fail 2004;6:593–9.

35. Damgaard M, Norsk P, Gustafsson F, et al. Hemodynamic and neuroendocrine responses to changes in sodium intake in compensated heart failure. Am J Physiol Regul Integr Comp Physiol 2006;290:R1294–301.

36. Nakasato M, Strunk CM, Guimaraes G, et al. Is the low-sodium diet actually indicated for all patients with stable heart failure? Arq Bras Cardiol 2010;94:86–94.

37. Hummel SL, Seymour EM, Brook RD, et al. Low-sodium DASH diet improves diastolic dysfunction and ventricular-arterial coupling in hypertensive heart failure with preserved ejection fraction. Circ Heart Fail 2013;6:1165–71.

38. Gupta D, Georgiopoulou VV, Kalogeropoulos A, et al. Dietary sodium intake in heart failure. Circulation 2012;126(4):479–85.

39. Goldsmith S. Hyponatremia in heart failure: time for a trial. J Card Fail 2013;19(6):398–400.

40. diNicholantonia JJ, Chatterjee S, O'Keefe JH. Dietary salt restriction in heart failure: where is the evidence? Prog Cardiovasc Dis 2016;58:401–6.

41. Filippatos TD, Elisaf MS. Hyponatremia in patients with heart failure. World J Cardiol 2013;5(9):317–28.

42. Konishi M, Haraguchi G, Ohigashi H, et al. Progression of hyponatremia is associated with increased cardiac mortality in patients hospitalized for acute decompensated heart failure. J Card Fail 2012;18:620–5.

43. Liamis G, Milionis H, Elisaf MS. A review of drug-induced hyponatremia. Am J Kidney Dis 2008;52:144–53.

Assessment of Volume Status Using Ultrasonography

Brooke A. Bailey, DNP, AGACNP, CNS*, Sarah Davis, DNP, AGACNP, FNP, Briana Witherspoon, DNP, APRN, ACNP

KEYWORDS

- Ultrasound • Ultrasonography • Volume status • Shock • Hypovolemia

KEY POINTS

- Critical care ultrasonography is useful in determining volume status in critically ill patients when the provider is trained and competent in the skill.
- Critical care ultrasonography leads to a prompt diagnosis and a more appropriate management of the critically ill patient.
- The increasing critical care patient population coupled with the shortage of critical care physicians amplifies the need for advanced practice providers to be competent in the management of critically ill patients.

INTRODUCTION

Assessment of volume status is fundamental when treating patients with hemodynamic instability.[1] The mean systemic filling pressure is decreased in an unstable, hemodynamic shock state resulting in an inadequate cardiac preload and cardiac output. This is present in hemodynamic instability caused by hypovolemia or vasodilation.[2] More importantly, a prolonged hypovolemic state decreases tissue perfusion, resulting in multiorgan dysfunction and organ failure, leading to increased mortality.[1,3] Many tools have been developed and used to evaluate and monitor volume status in patients with hemodynamic instability, but most are invasive and not without risk.[1]

Ultrasonography is a noninvasive modality that can be used to evaluate volume status in critically ill patients. When combined with the clinical examination, critical care ultrasonography can lead to prompt diagnosis and help guide treatment in critically ill patients with hemodynamic instability. Critical care ultrasonography is convenient, safe, and useful when evaluating volume status in the critically ill patient population. It consists of 2 examinations: general critical care ultrasonography and basic critical

Disclosure statement: The authors have no conflicts of interest.
Department of Advanced Practice, Vanderbilt University Medical Center, 1161 21st Avenue South, AA-1214 Medical Center North, Nashville, TN 37232, USA
* Corresponding author.
E-mail address: brooke.a.bailey@vanderbilt.edu

Nurs Clin N Am 52 (2017) 269–279
http://dx.doi.org/10.1016/j.cnur.2017.01.004
0029-6465/17/© 2017 Elsevier Inc. All rights reserved.
nursing.theclinics.com

care echocardiography.[4] The general critical care ultrasonography examination involves assessment and evaluation of the lungs, pleura, abdomen, and vasculature, whereas the basic critical care echocardiogram involves evaluation of the heart and inferior vena cava (IVC).[4] Additionally, ultrasonography can be used for procedural guidance to decrease the risk of complications.[5]

BACKGROUND

Ultrasonography was introduced to medicine in the 1950s.[6] At this time, machines were large and stationary, limiting the usability and accessibility of most populations within the acute setting, including patients requiring intensive care. Large, bulky ultrasound machines were difficult to transfer let alone be taken to the bedside of critically ill patients in intensive care unit rooms where there were space restraints. These restraints prevented rapid evaluation with ultrasonography. With the advancements of technology, ultrasound machines are now small, portable, and easy to transfer to the patient's bedside to evaluate and manage the patient's condition promptly.[6,7]

Historically, ultrasound examinations were limited to the subspecialties of obstetrics, cardiology, radiology, and anesthesiology, until the 1990s when ultrasonography use expanded to include emergency medicine. The Focused Assessment with Sonography for Trauma (FAST) examination was developed and used within emergency medicine to assess trauma patients for hemopericardium and hemoperitoneums.[6] The efficiency, accuracy, and rapid access allowed evaluation of specific trauma conditions, which in turn decreased hospital length of stay, treatment costs, time to definitive diagnosis or operation, and mortality.[8,9]

Emergency medicine ultrasonography curriculum and Emergency Ultrasound Guidelines have since been developed and published by the Society of Academic Emergency Medicine.[6] Recently, the Society of Critical Care Medicine has incorporated ultrasonography examination into recommended routine evaluation of the critically ill patient. It is used to assess and interpret imaging promptly and manage the patient condition leading to improved treatment options and plans.[5]

In 2009, the American College of Chest Physicians and La Société de Réanimation de Langue Française published the consensus statement for critical care ultrasonography, which led to the international expert statement on training standards.[10,11] Use of ultrasonography in the critical care population allows providers to assess and interpret imaging in real time, providing a more prompt diagnosis and management of potentially life-threatening conditions. Ultrasonography has evolved from minimal use among a select group of medical specialties to guiding and directing the management of the most acutely ill patients within emergency and critical care medicine.[5]

IMPORTANCE

The American College of Chest Physicians and La Société de Réanimation de Langue Française consensus statement on critical care ultrasonography includes 2 focused examinations: a general critical care ultrasonography examination and a basic critical care echocardiogram. The general critical care ultrasonography examination includes evaluation of the lungs, pleura, abdomen, and vasculature. The basic critical care echocardiogram includes the evaluation of the heart and IVC. The consensus statement recommends that all critical care providers be trained and competent in general critical care ultrasonography and basic echocardiography.[11]

Traditionally, physicians were the sole providers using ultrasonography in practice. As a result of the growing population and increase in acuity of critically ill patients, advanced practice providers, including nurse practitioners and physician assistants, are being trained in using ultrasonography to evaluate and treat patients in emergency and critical care medicine.[12–14] As advanced practice providers embark on using ultrasonography in practice, it is important to show competence. A recent study involving nurse practitioners practicing in the emergency department evaluated 5 nurse practitioners after ultrasonography training. Instruction included a 2-day, 16-hour course and supervision from emergency medicine physicians for 1 year. After training, ultrasound examinations were logged over a 2-month period and reviewed by an expert. Results showed a 93% sensitivity and 98% specificity in nurse practitioners correctly interpreting ultrasound imaging. Although this study only included 5 nurse practitioners, the study was able to show the advanced skill set advanced practice providers encompass in the management of the critically ill.[15]

General critical care ultrasonography and basic critical care echocardiography have become first-line diagnostic tools for providers managing acute medical conditions in the emergency and critical care setting.[10,16] Ultrasonography examinations are performed and interpreted by the provider at the patient's bedside, making results immediately available, and the examination can be repeated as often as needed to evaluate response to therapy. Ultrasound findings should be combined with the patient's history of present illness, physical examination, and laboratory and diagnostic study results for the most accurate diagnosis and appropriate management.[17] By using ultrasonography at the bedside, time to diagnosis, health care costs, radiation exposure, time to definitive operation, hospital length of stay, and mortality all decrease.[4,8–10,16] Ultrasonography also personalize the patient care experience.[4] Health care costs decrease when ultrasonography is used because of avoidance of expensive and invasive diagnostic tools.[1]

Lung ultrasonography has been shown to be 78% to 91% specific in the diagnosis of a pneumothorax while only identified 30% to 72% of the time on chest radiographs.[18] Ultrasonography is now considered a superior diagnostic tool when evaluating common pathologic conditions when compared with chest radiography.[19] Patient exposure to radiation decreases when ultrasonography is used because of the decreased number of chest radiographs and computed tomography scans ordered.[16] Outcomes also improve when used for procedural guidance.[4] Ultrasonography is useful in a variety of critical care conditions leading to prompt diagnosis of life-threatening conditions while guiding management in critically ill patients.

ASSESSMENT OF VOLUME STATUS VIA ULTRASONOGRAPHY
General Critical Care Ultrasonography Examination

Lung and pleural ultrasonography
Lung and pleural ultrasonography is useful in contributing to the assessment of volume status and a variety of other life-threatening conditions such as pneumothorax and acute respiratory distress syndrome. When evaluating the lungs and pleura, the provider should evaluate the lungs in a step-by-step approach and be able to identify A lines, B lines, lung sliding, lung tissue appearance, and the presence of pleural effusions.[20]

Lung and pleural ultrasonography is performed by using either the phased-array transducer (3.5–5 MHz) or the linear array transducer (7.5–10 MHz). When using the phased-array transducer, the marker is pointed cephalad while the linear array transducer is pointed to 9 o'clock. Some providers prefer the linear array transducer during the anterior view evaluation because of the higher frequency imaging of the pleural line when evaluating lung sliding. The patient is positioned sitting up when possible, but typically in critically ill patients this proves to be a challenge, defaulting to the patient being in the supine position. When evaluating the lungs and pleura, the anterior, lateral, and posterior lung fields are assessed for A lines, B lines, lung sliding, lung tissue appearance, and pleural effusions. The provider starts the examination by scanning anterior lung fields with either the phased-array or linear-array transducer. The probe is placed adjacent to the sternum on either the left or right at the second or third intercostal place. The provider scans down each intercostal space while evaluating for A lines, B lines, lung sliding, and lung tissue appearance. The lateral and posterior lung fields are then evaluated using the phased-array transducer because of the deeper views that can be obtained. Again, A lines, B lines, lung tissue appearance, and lung sliding are assessed in addition to the presence of pleural effusions. Assessment of the lateral and posterior lung fields for pleural effusions requires the provider be able to locate the diaphragm, chest wall, and lung. Once these boundaries are located, the space is evaluated for any hypoechoic fluid to determine the presence of a pleural effusion.[21,22] The examination is then repeated on the opposite side.

When evaluating the lungs via ultrasonography, A lines are an expected physiologic finding. They are equally spaced horizontal lines, which demonstrate normal aerated lung. Conversely, B lines are cone-shaped artifacts that extend the full length of the ultrasound screen.[22] B lines can represent abnormal physiology if 2 or more are seen in a lone view and require further inquiry. Differential diagnoses when more than 2 B-lines are present include pulmonary edema, acute respiratory distress syndrome, pneumonia, and pulmonary fibrosis.[20] Although pneumonia and acute respiratory distress syndrome cannot be ruled out, pulmonary edema is the more likely diagnosis if B lines are present bilaterally and can contribute to the evaluation of volume status.[20] Extravascular lung water volume greater than 500 mL has also been found to be associated with pulmonary edema.[23] A study by Agricola and colleagues[23] found lung ultrasonography to be 90% sensitive and 86% specific when identifying extravascular lung water volume greater than 500 mL.[23] A prospective, cross-sectional study on resident physicians novice to lung ultrasonography looked at identification and interpretation of B lines. It was reported they were able to identify B lines after a 30-minute lung ultrasonography training session. There was an 80% sensitivity and specificity compared with experts, proving that training can be prompt and competency reasonably easy to obtain.[20]

The identification of pleural effusions can be an indication of a hypervolemic state, answering the inquiry of a patient's volume status,[24] which can be helpful when evaluating heart failure patients and can guide diuretic therapy.[25] When assessing for pleural effusions, pleural ultrasonography is superior compared with chest radiography.[17] A study by Rozycki and colleagues[26] found 84% sensitivity, 100% specificity, and 94% accuracy when pleural ultrasonography was used to identify pleural effusions. Lung and pleural ultrasonography is quick and easy to train, resulting in prompt diagnoses and management in critically ill patients. It is a 1C recommendation.[27]

Abdominal ultrasonography

Abdominal ultrasonography is useful in evaluating a patient's volume status while also being able to diagnose multiple potential shock states associated with free fluid.[28] Abdominal ultrasonography is performed with the patient in a supine position. A general phased-array or curved phased-array, low-frequency transducer is used during this examination. The most common ultrasonography examination used to evaluate the abdomen is the FAST examination. The FAST examination evaluates the abdominal, pelvic, and pericardial space for free fluid. During this examination, the transducer is placed in the subcostal 4-chamber position under the patient's xiphoid. The ultrasound is set to an abdominal examination setting, and the marker is directed toward the patient's right shoulder. After evaluating the pericardial space, the marker is moved to the right lateral position with the marker pointed cephalad to evaluate the hepatorenal space, kidney, and pleural space. The transducer is then moved to the left lateral position to evaluate the splenorenal space, kidney, and pleural space. The abdomen is also assessed for peritoneal fluid with the transducer placed on the right and left midabdomen to evaluate for free fluid. The last area in the FAST examination is the pelvis. The bladder and vesicouterine space in females or rectovesicular space in males is assessed for free fluid. The transducer is placed superior to the pelvic bone to obtain these views. Any hypoechoic fluid noted during the examination is concerning for free fluid and should be evaluated further.[28]

The FAST examination has been useful for guidance in management of hemorrhagic shock with an abdominal or pelvic origin.[28] Within the trauma population, this examination is found to decrease treatment costs, hospital length of stay, time to operation, and mortality.[8,9] A randomized controlled trial by Melniker and colleagues[8] found that by using point-of-care limited ultrasonography on trauma patients, time to definitive operation when compared with the control group was 64% less.[8] Fewer computed tomography scans were ordered, and hospital length of stay decreased, fewer complications occurred, and health care costs decreased by 35%.[8]

Vasculature

Although the vascular ultrasound examination can be useful in identifying or ruling out deep venous thrombosis in the lower extremities, it is not routinely used to evaluate volume status unlike lung, pleural, and abdominal ultrasonography. Xing and colleagues[29] found a unique measurement that correlates to invasive central venous pressure measurements.[29] This study found that measurement from the point the internal jugular vein collapses to the center of the right atrium in the apical 4-chamber view via ultrasonography can be calculated to correlate to central venous pressures. Once this distance is measured in centimeters, it is converted to a central venous pressure value (1.36 cm H_2O = 1 mm Hg).[29] Although not used routinely at this time, this could be another safe, noninvasive approach to evaluate volume status in critically ill patients.

Basic Critical Care Echocardiography

In additional to general critical care ultrasonography, basic critical care echocardiography is a skill routinely used by trained providers to evaluate volume status in critically ill patients. It can also be used to evaluate for life-threatening disease processes and differentiate between various shock states including hypovolemic, distributive, cardiogenic, and obstructive shock.[3,17] A critical care provider trained in basic critical care echocardiography should be competent in identifying critical, life-threatening conditions. These include severe hypovolemia, left and right ventricular failure, cardiac tamponade, acute massive left-sided valvular regurgitation, and cardiac arrest.[11]

In addition to identifying life-threatening conditions, the provider should be competent in evaluating the left and right ventricles, pericardial space, IVC, and cardiac valves.[11] When examining the ventricles, the left ventricle contractile pattern and bilateral ventricle size and systolic function are evaluated. The pericardial space is assessed for the presence of an effusion and any evidence of cardiac tamponade. On visualization of the IVC, size and respiratory variability are evaluated.[11] Color Doppler can be used during assessment of the valves to evaluate for severe valvular regurgitation.[11] Each abnormality identified can help to rule in or rule out a diagnosis and lead to prompt management.

To prepare for a basic critical care echocardiogram, the patient is positioned in the left lateral decubitus position, as most cardiac views are optimized in this position.

This is true apart from the subcostal views in which the patient is positioned supine. The phased-array transducer is used during this examination with the ultrasound machine set to the cardiac mode.[30]

The parasternal long-axis view is obtained by placing the transducer between the third and fifth intercostal space alongside the patient's left sternum. The marker on the ultrasound transducer is pointed to the patient's right shoulder. To obtain the parasternal short-axis view, the transducer is turned 90° clockwise from the parasternal long-axis view position. The transducer marker is then pointed toward the patient's left shoulder. The apical 4-chamber view is obtained by placing the transducer infero-lateral to the patient's left nipple. The marker is pointed to approximately 3 o'clock. The patient is then positioned supine for the subcostal long-axis 4-chamber and IVC views. The transducer is positioned inferior to the xiphoid process with the marker directed toward the patient's left shoulder. The subcostal IVC longitudinal view can then be obtained by rotating the transducer counterclockwise with the marker pointed cephalad.[7,30] If the subcostal IVC view is unobtainable, another approach when assessing the IVC is the transhepatic, lateral view.[17]

When specifically assessing for volume status, it is recommended to obtain all 5 cardiac views:

- Parasternal long-axis
- Parasternal short-axis
- Apical 4-chamber
- Subcostal long-axis 4-chamber
- Subcostal IVC longitudinal.[17]

These views allow the provider to have a comprehensive understanding of the patient's presenting condition. Many findings throughout the examination can help determine volume status: ejection fraction, left ventricle function, the presence of a pericardial effusion, compare right and left ventricle size, and determine size and variability of the IVC.[17] A qualitative assessment of the ejection fraction and left ventricle wall function can be evaluated throughout all cardiac views during the basic critical care echocardiogram apart from the subcostal IVC view.[17]

The apical 4-chamber view is superior when comparing the size of the right and left ventricles, which should be no greater than a ratio of 0.6:1.[3,17] Evaluation of the pericardial space to assess for an effusion can be obtained in the parasternal long-axis, apical 4-chamber, and subcostal 4-chamber views. The subcostal IVC view is superior in determining preload sensitivity on viewing the IVC.[17] However, the main evaluation of volume status is determined by the IVC assessment. Once volume status is determined, the remaining basic critical care echocardiogram findings help lead to a diagnosis and guide management.

Once the IVC is identified in the subcostal view, the provider confirms the IVC by following it into the right atrium. The IVC can then be measured. There are 2 common measurement strategies. The first strategy involves calculating the caval index and the measurement of the IVC. The caval index is the difference in the maximum and minimum diameter of the IVC during the respiratory cycle divided by the expiratory diameter multiplied by 100.[31] The maximal IVC diameter is measured upon expiration, whereas the minimal IVC diameter is measured upon inspiration.[31] A 50% caval index correlates to a central venous pressure of 8 mm Hg.[32] A change in IVC diameter of 15% or more after fluid resuscitation in mechanically ventilated patients suggests preload responsiveness.[27] The second measurement is of the IVC diameter directly before it enters the right atrium. An IVC diameter less than 2 cm, with a respiratory variability greater than 50% during inspiration compares with a central venous pressure measurement of 10 mm Hg or less, whereas a measurement greater than 2 cm, with a respiratory variability less than 50% compares with a central venous pressure more than 10 mm Hg.[3]

A few studies suggested that assessment of the IVC via ultrasonography is adequate for the evaluation of volume status.[33–35] Although this is true, most of those study populations comprised patients with severe sepsis or septic shock who were mechanically ventilated.[33–35] Thus, this assessment is not completely generalizable to all critical care populations. A prospective clinical study by Barbier and colleagues[33] collected data from 33 mechanically ventilated patients with sepsis related to an acute lung injury. Change in IVC diameter and cardiac index after fluid resuscitation was found to be strongly related, thus concluding that change in IVC diameter via ultrasonography is a reliable tool to assess fluid responsiveness in mechanically ventilated septic patients. Another prospective clinical study by Feissel and colleagues[34] collected data from mechanically ventilated patients with a diagnosis of septic shock. This study compared IVC diameter change and cardiac output. It validated that change in IVC diameter via ultrasonography is an adequate tool to assess fluid responsiveness. In another study by Schefold and colleagues,[35] assessment of IVC change in diameter via ultrasonography was again found to be an adequate tool to evaluate fluid status in mechanically ventilated, severe sepsis, and septic shock patients. Although most studies have evaluated mechanically ventilated patients with sepsis, a study by de Valk and colleagues[31] looked at spontaneous breathing patients with undifferentiated shock. This prospective, cross-sectional observational study found that a caval index less than 36.5% predicted inadequate fluid resuscitation. A higher caval index of greater than 36.5% did not predict adequate fluid responsiveness. This could have been because of the spontaneous breathing patient population studied.[31] More studies looking at spontaneous breathing patients and change in diameter of IVC during a shock state are needed to determine IVC assessment via ultrasonography. By measuring the IVC via ultrasonography, volume status can be immediately determined and replaced, even if central venous access is not immediately available.[27] Assessment of preload responsiveness via basic echocardiogram in mechanically ventilated patients is a 1B recommendation.[27]

Another study focusing on undifferentiated shock favored ultrasonography as a routine, first-line diagnostic tool to evaluate critically ill patients' volume status.[36] A prospective observational study by Weekes and colleagues[36] evaluated left ventricular function and measured caval index in 24 patients with shock to determine fluid responsiveness. The study found that a persistent decrease in caval index measurements after fluid resuscitation was more likely associated with cardiac dysfunction and concern for cardiogenic shock.[36] By using such knowledge, the provider can narrow diagnoses of the presenting, undifferentiated shock state by examining the left ventricular function and IVC via ultrasonography.[36]

A randomized controlled trial by Jones and colleagues[37] showed that by incorporating basic critical care echocardiography into a protocol for undifferentiated hypotension, differential diagnoses narrow more rapidly.[37] Patient diagnoses, when evaluated with ultrasonography at the time of presentation, were 80% correct at 15 minutes, whereas the control group with just the standard of care diagnostic workup diagnosed 50% correctly at 15 minutes. The list of differential diagnoses narrows more rapidly when ultrasonography is used in patients with undifferentiated shock.[37] A variety of focused ultrasound protocols have been proposed within the literature to help guide providers in a thorough ultrasound evaluation in patients with shock.[3,38]

Multiple studies have found ultrasound valuable specifically in patients with hemorrhagic shock.[39,40] A prospective, control study by Akilli and colleagues[39] showed that evaluation of the IVC in patients with acute blood loss is more predictable than other noninvasive measurements such as heart rate, blood pressure, serum lactate, and base deficit. In hemorrhagic shock, an ultrasound examination and can help predict 24-hour mortality from initial time of presentation.[39] Although a small prospective study with only 30 participants, Yanagawa and colleagues[40] found that ultrasound findings of a decreased IVC diameter in trauma patients was a more valuable predictor of hemorrhagic shock reoccurring than blood pressure, calling for further investigation and need for additional interventions.

In patients with acute heart failure, basic critical care echocardiography is useful in evaluation of volume status and guides diuretic therapy in the inpatient and outpatient setting.[20] Multiple studies on outpatient heart failure concluded that management is more appropriate when a basic, goal-directed echocardiogram is combined with standard signs and symptoms of acute heart failure (eg, daily weights, peripheral edema, acute heart failure symptoms, laboratory test results). It was concluded that assessment of IVC and pleural cavities via ultrasonography significantly increased prediction of diuretic management in outpatient heart failure patients.[25] Basic critical care echocardiography aids to diagnose and guide management of critically ill patients and is especially useful in determining volume status of hemodynamically unstable patients. Once the initial, basic echocardiogram examination is complete, it can be routinely repeated to evaluate response to therapy, guide future management, and monitor progression of the disease.[17]

GUIDELINES FOR CRITICAL CARE ULTRASONOGRAPHY TRAINING

Guidelines for critical care ultrasonography training were established at the at the 23rd European Society of Intensive Care Medicine and based on the American College of Chest Physicians and La Société de Réanimation de Langue Française critical care ultrasonography consensus statement.[10] Training guidelines recommend 10 hours of training for general critical care ultrasonography and an additional 10 hours in basic critical care echocardiography. Both didactic and image-based training is recommended with options of both traditional lecturing and internet-based education. Training should include hands-on opportunities on normal volunteers to learn how to manipulate the transducer, become familiar with standard views, and adapt to spatial orientation. Faculty should include providers formerly trained who routinely use ultrasonography in practice.[10]

LIMITATIONS

There are several limitations when performing a general critical care ultrasonography examination and basic critical care echocardiogram. The critically ill patient population can be erratic and unpredictable. When evaluating volume status in critically ill patients, assessment may be difficult because of a patient's spontaneous respirations, body habitus, a thrombus or mass obstructing the vasculature, incisions, bulky dressings, central venous line catheters, chest tubes, abdominal or chest drains, and any other equipment or monitoring that can obscure ultrasound views.[29] A patient's hemodynamic instability or timing of a needed examination can also deter the provider from ultrasonography evaluation.[29]

Another significant limitation includes provider training and competence in ultrasonography. For a general critical care ultrasonography examination and basic critical care echocardiogram imaging and interpretation to be accurate, the provider must be competent in the skill. Competency requires specific training and practice in critical care ultrasonography.[4] Many organizations provide training that meets the critical care ultrasonography training recommendations published by the American College of Chest Physicians and La Société de Réanimation de Langue Française. Although many organizations provide this training, it can be costly, time consuming, and require travel. We suggest that larger institutions develop in-network training on critical care ultrasonography for all providers managing critically ill patients. Although it is recommended the provider be competent in critical care ultrasonography before diagnosing independently, guidelines do not give specific requirements for competency; therefore, competence is determined by each individual institution.[11]

Limitations regarding studies reviewed for this article include small sample sizes and lack of multi-institution involvement. Another limitation is the lack of studies on advanced practice provider training and competency in ultrasonography. Many areas of focus need additional research. Ultrasonography use for assessment of volume status is supported by the literature, and recommendations range from 1B to 2C.[27]

SUMMARY

Critical care ultrasonography is useful in determining volume status in critically ill patients when the provider is trained and competent in the skill. Critical care ultrasonography leads to a prompt diagnosis and a more appropriate management of the critically ill patient. The increasing critical care patient population coupled with the shortage of critical care physicians amplifies the need for advanced practice providers to be competent in the management of critically ill patients. Ultrasonography in critical care decreases health care costs, time to diagnosis, hospital length of stay, time to definitive operation, and mortality.[8,9] It also has the potential to improve patient and family satisfaction by involving them during the examination. By performing critical care ultrasonography, the heart, lungs, pleura, abdomen, and vasculature are evaluated, allowing more efficient patient management and ultimately improving patient outcomes.

REFERENCES

1. Szopinski J, Kusza K, Semionow M. Microcirculatory responses to hypovolemic shock. J Trauma 2011;71(6):1779–88.
2. Boulain T, Cecconi M. Can one size fit all? The fine line between fluid overload and hypovolemia. Intensive Care Med 2015;41(3):544.
3. Perera P, Mailhot T, Riley D, et al. The RUSH exam: Rapid Ultrasound in SHock in the evaluation of the critically ill. Emerg Med Clin North Am 2010;28(1):29–56.
4. Coleman NE, Slonim AD. Ultrasound in critical care medicine: improving patient care and reducing cost. In: Levitov AB, Mayo PH, Slonim AD, editors. Critical care ultrasonography. 2nd edition. New York: McGraw Hill Education; 2014. p. 3–7.
5. Morris AE. Point-of-care ultrasound: seeing the future. Curr Probl Diagn Radiol 2015;44(1):3–7.
6. Kendall JL, Hoffenberg SR, Smith S. History of emergency and critical care ultrasound: the evolution of a new imaging paradigm. Crit Care Med 2007;35(5): S126–30.
7. Royse CF, Canty DJ, Faris J, et al. Core review: physician-performed ultrasound: the time has come for routine use in acute care medicine. Anesth Analg 2012; 115(5):1007–28.
8. Melniker LA, Leibner E, McKenney MG, et al. Randomized controlled clinical trial of point-of-care, limited ultrasonography for trauma in the emergency department: the first sonography outcomes assessment program trial. Ann Emerg Med 2006;48(3):227–35.

9. Blood CG, Puyana JC, Pitlyk PJ, et al. An assessment of the potential for reducing future combat deaths through medical technologies and training. J Trauma 2002; 53(6):1160–5.

10. Cholley BP. International expert statement on training standards for critical care ultrasonography. Intensive Care Med 2011;37:1077–83.

11. Mayo PH, Beaulieu Y, Doelken P, et al. American College of Chest Physicians/La Société de Réanimation de Langue Française statement on competence in critical care ultrasonography. Chest 2009;135(4):1050–60.

12. Halpern NA, Pastores SM. Critical care medicine in the United States 2000-2005: an analysis of bed numbers, occupancy rate, payer mix, and costs. Crit Care Med 2010;38(1):65–71.

13. Angus DC, Kelley MA, Schmitz RJ, et al. Current and projected workforce requirements for care of the critically ill and patients with pulmonary disease: can we meet the requirements of an aging population? JAMA 2000;284(21):2762–70.

14. Fry M. Literature review of the impact of nurse practitioners in critical care services. Nurs Crit Care 2011;16(2):58–66.

15. Henderson SO, Ahern T, Williams D, et al. Emergency department ultrasound by nurse practitioners. J Am Acad Nurse Pract 2016;22:352–5.

16. Levitov A, Mayo PH, Slonim AD. Critical care ultrasonography. Ultrasound Med Biol 2014;39(11):2211.

17. Koenig S, Narasimhan M, Mayo PH. Goal-directed echocardiography in the ICU. In: Levitov AB, Mayo PH, Slonim AD, editors. Critical care ultrasonography. 2nd edition. New York: McGraw Hill Education; 2014. p. 57–63.

18. Ioos V, Galbois A, Chalumeau-Lemoine L, et al. An integrated approach for prescribing fewer chest x-rays in the ICU. Ann Intensive Care 2011;1(1):4.

19. Xirouchaki N, Magkanas E, Vaporidi K, et al. Lung ultrasound in critically ill patients: comparison with bedside chest radiography. Intensive Care Med 2011; 37:1488–93.

20. Cheim AT, Chan CH, Ander DS, et al. Comparison of expert and novice sonographers' performance in focused lung ultrasonography in dyspnea (FLUID) to diagnose patients with acute heart failure syndrome. Acad Emerg Med 2015;22(5): 564–73.

21. Eisen L, Doelken P, Ahmad S. Ultrasound evaluation of the pleura. In: Levitov AB, Mayo PH, Slonim AD, editors. Critical care ultrasonography. 2nd edition. New York: McGraw Hill Education; 2014. p. 197–206.

22. Kory P, Mayo PH. Ultrasound evaluation of the lung. In: Levitov AB, Mayo PH, Slonim AD, editors. Critical care ultrasonography. 2nd edition. New York: McGraw Hill Education; 2014. p. 207–17.

23. Agricola E, Bove T, Oppizzi M, et al. "Ultrasound comet-tail images": a marker of pulmonary edema: a comparative study with wedge pressure and extravascular lung water. Chest 2005;127(5):1690–5.

24. Weintraub NL, Collins SP, Pang PS, et al. Acute heart failure syndromes: emergency department presentation, treatment, and disposition: current approaches and future aims: a scientific statement from the American heart association. Circulation 2010;122:1975–96.

25. Gunderson GH, Norekval RM, Haug HH, et al. Adding point of care ultrasound to assess volume status in heart failure patients in a nurse-led outpatient clinic. A randomized study. Heart 2016;102:29–34.

26. Rozycki GS, Pennington SD, Feliciano DV. Surgeon-performed ultrasound in the critical care setting: its use as an extension of the physical examination to detect pleural effusion. J Trauma 2001;50(4):636–42.

27. Levitov A, Frankel HL, Blaivas M, et al. Guidelines for the appropriate use of bedside general and cardiac ultrasonography in the evaluation of critically Ill Patients—Part II: cardiac ultrasonography. Crit Care Med 2016;44(6):1206–27.
28. Shaves SC, Frankel HL. Ultrasound evaluation of the abdomen. In: Levitov AB, Mayo PH, Slonim AD, editors. Critical care ultrasonography. 2nd edition. New York: McGraw Hill Education; 2014. p. 219–33.
29. Xing C, Liu Y, Zhao M, et al. New method for noninvasive quantification of central venous pressure by ultrasound. Circ Cardiovasc Imaging 2015;8(5):e003085.
30. Cardenas-Garcia J, Mayo PH. Transthoracic echocardiography: image acquisition. In: Levitov AB, Mayo PH, Slonim AD, editors. Critical care ultrasonography. 2nd edition. New York: McGraw Hill Education; 2014. p. 65–75.
31. de Valk S, Olgers TJ, Holman M, et al. The caval index: an adequate non-invasive ultrasound parameter to predict fluid responsiveness in the emergency department? BMC Anesthesiol 2014;14(1):114.
32. Nagdev AD, Merchant RC, Tirado-Gonzalez A, et al. Emergency department bedside ultrasonographic measurement of the caval index for noninvasive determination of low central venous pressure. Ann Emerg Med 2010;55(3):290–5.
33. Barbier C, Loubières Y, Schmit C, et al. Respiratory changes in inferior vena cava diameter are helpful in predicting fluid responsiveness in ventilated septic patients. Intensive Care Med 2004;30(9):1740–6.
34. Feissel M, Michard F, Faller JP, et al. The respiratory variation in inferior vena cava diameter as a guide to fluid therapy. Intensive Care Med 2004;30(9):1834–7.
35. Schefold JC, Storm C, Bercker S, et al. Inferior vena cava diameter correlates with invasive hemodynamic measures in mechanically ventilated intensive care unit patients with sepsis. J Emerg Med 2010;38(5):632–7.
36. Weekes AJ, Tassone HM, Babcock A, et al. Comparison of serial qualitative and quantitative assessments of caval index and left ventricular systolic function during early fluid resuscitation of hypotensive emergency department patients. Acad Emerg Med 2011;18(9):912–21.
37. Jones AE, Tayal VS, Sullivan DM, et al. Randomized, controlled trial of immediate versus delayed goal-directed ultrasound to identify the cause of nontraumatic hypotension in emergency department patients. Crit Care Med 2004;32(8):1703–8.
38. Atkinson PRT, McAuley DJ, Kendall RJ, et al. Abdominal and Cardiac Evaluation with Sonography in Shock (ACES): an approach by emergency physicians for the use of ultrasound in patients with undifferentiated hypotension. Emerg Med J 2009;26(2):87–91.
39. Akilli B, Bayir A, Kara F, et al. Inferior vena cava diameter as a marker of early hemorrhagic shock: a comparative study. Ulus Travma Acil Cerrahi Derg 2010; 16(2):113–8.
40. Yanagawa Y, Sakamoto T, Okada Y. Hypovolemic shock evaluated by sonographic measurement of the inferior vena cava during resuscitation in trauma patients. J Trauma 2007;63(6):1245–8.

Metabolic and Electrolyte Abnormalities Related to Use of Bowel in Urologic Reconstruction

 CrossMark

Amanda N. Squiers, DNP, APRN, ANP-BC, GNP-BC[a,b,*],
Karleena Twitchell, MN, APRN[a,c]

KEYWORDS

- Metabolic • Electrolyte • Bowel • Urologic reconstruction

KEY POINTS

- Use of bowel in urologic reconstruction can result in acid-base and electrolyte abnormalities.
- Severity can vary based on type of segment, length of segment, and contact time with urine.
- Patients with impairment in renal or hepatic function are at greatest risk

INTRODUCTION

There is a long history of the utilization of bowel segments for urologic reconstructive surgery. The first known urinary diversion using the intestine was accomplished in 1851 by Sir John Simon, with the completion of the first urinary colic fistula.[1] This initial procedure led to the development of a variety of techniques using autologous bowel for urinary diversion and bladder augmentation. Since that time, there has been a growing understanding to the potential electrolyte and metabolic complications associated with the utilization of bowel in urologic reconstruction. These complications depend on a variety of factors, including the length and type of bowel segment used for the reconstruction, and the amount of time that urine is in contact with the

The authors have nothing to disclose.
[a] Oregon Health Science University School of Nursing, 3455 Southwest US Veterans Hospital Road, Portland, OR 97239, USA; [b] Department of Urologic Surgery, Oregon Health Science University School of Medicine, 3455 Southwest US Veterans Hospital Road, Portland, OR 97239, USA; [c] Division of Cardiac and Surgical Subspecialty Critical Care, Department of Anesthesiology, Oregon Health Science University School of Medicine, 3455 Southwest US Veterans Hospital Road, Portland, OR 97239, USA
* Corresponding author. 3455 Southwest US Veterans Hospital Road, Portland, OR 97239.
E-mail address: squiersa@ohsu.edu

bowel segment.[2] These primary factors can also be affected by several patient comorbidities, including hepatic and renal insufficiency. The most common acute and chronic complications of these procedures include metabolic acidosis or alkalosis, electrolyte imbalance, malabsorption of vitamins, abnormalities in bone metabolism, abnormal drug absorption, and formation of renal and bladder calculi. This article reviews the types of urologic reconstructions and their potential metabolic and electrolyte complications that result from the use of gastrointestinal segments in these surgeries.

RECONSTRUCTION: INDICATIONS AND TYPES

The goal of a urinary diversion or augmentation is to create a method for urine storage and elimination when the bladder is impaired either structurally, functionally, or as a result of malignancy. The most common indications for urologic reconstruction are:

- Bladder cancer
- Other malignancies in the pelvis that require removal of the bladder
- Congenital bladder abnormalities
- Bladder dysfunction (ie, neurogenic bladder)
- Bladder trauma

Depending on underlying pathologic condition, patients may undergo urinary diversion with an orthotopic neobladder, continent cutaneous diversion, or conduit. The neobladder most closely resembles the natural bladder's function. Although techniques may vary, it often consists of ileum or colon segments that are detubularized and folded in different variations to form the neobladder that is then connected to the native urethra.[2] A continent cutaneous diversion is a similar procedure to the formation of a neobladder, with the exception of the creation of a catheterizable channel that is brought to the skin surface on the abdomen. This form of urinary diversion requires the patient to be able to catheterize a stoma. Finally, the conduit is the most commonly used type of urinary diversion.[2] It involves taking the ends of the ureters and anastomosing them to a segment of small bowel, most commonly ileum, which forms a conduit to the skin surface. Urine then drains through the ostomy into a bag on the patient's abdomen. These types of diversions may be performed for structural impairment, functional impairment, or cancer.

In contrast to a diversion, patients may undergo augmentation of their native bladder known as cystoplasty. The procedure involves opening the bladder and suturing on a segment of bowel.[3] For this procedure, cecum, colon, or stomach may be used but ileum is the most common segment. This procedure is reserved for patients with either a low capacity bladder or those who store urine under high pressure.

COMPLICATIONS RELATED TO BOWEL IN URINARY TRACT

Severity of metabolic and electrolyte derangements arising from use of bowel in the urinary tract can vary based on several factors: contact time with urine, underlying renal or hepatic dysfunction, and what type of bowel is used. Potential complications are best understood by considering the original function of the bowel segment that is used. Transport of water across bowel segments follows the osmotic gradient and depends on intracellular junctions.[4] Although gastric mucosa offers the least absorptive properties, absorption decreases antegrade as it moves from the jejunum, which has the highest absorption, to the colon, which has the least.[5] The absorptive ability is related to the decreased permeability of the tight junctions moving from jejunum to colon.[6] Here, abnormalities are broken down by type of bowel segment that is interposed in the urinary tract and discussed in detail. The nonspecific symptoms these patients may present with are listed in **Table 1**.

Gastric

Use of stomach in urinary reconstruction can have benefit over other segments in select populations. The first potential benefit in using gastric mucosa is related to the tight junctions between cells, which do not have the same type absorptive properties of other segments. Second, when the gastric mucosa is relocated to the urinary tract it continues to secrete hydrochloric acid, which is thought to reduce bacterial colonization, urinary tract infections, and stones common to other segments.[7] Also, patients who undergo gastrocystoplasty do not have the same issues with mucus production commonly seen with other segments, which can contribute to impaired drainage of catheters and stone formation. Finally, it has potential benefit in patients with metabolic acidosis. First recommended by Adams and colleagues[8] for this population, gastric segments offer benefit in secretion of acid with increase in serum bicarbonate, which can benefit patients with underlying metabolic acidosis.

Despite these benefits, stomach is not the perfect urologic substitute. Patients who have undergone gastrocystoplasty are at particular risk for hypokalemic hypochloremic metabolic alkalosis.[6] This is related to the hydrogen potassium (H+/K+) antiport, which secretes hydrogen ions in exchange for potassium.[9] The secreted hydrogen ion comes from the breakdown of carbonic acid, which results in systemic release of bicarbonate. The excess bicarbonate ion is then excreted into the urine. However, if renal impairment is present, bicarbonate excretion is impaired and subsequent

Table 1
Signs and Symptoms of Potential Metabolic Complications

Metabolic & Electrolyte Disorders	Signs & Symptoms
Metabolic acidosis[26] • Jejunum, ileum, colon	Hyperpnea and Kussmaul respirations Headache Lethargy Stupor
Metabolic alkalosis[26] • Gastric	Mental confusion Obtundation Seizures Paresthesias Muscle cramping Tetany Arrhythmias
Vitamin B12 deficiency[28] • Gastric, ileum, colon	Anemia Weight loss Diarrhea or constipation Glossitis Jaundice Neuropathy Paresthesia Muscle weakness
Hyperchloremia[29] • Ileum, colon	Dry mucous membranes Coated tongue No axillary sweat Hypotension Tachycardia

potassium wasting results.[9] This can be exacerbated during times of dehydration. These complications have led to decreased use of gastrocystoplasty in patients with renal insufficiency.

Metabolic alkalosis may be further compounded if hypergastrinemia is present. Gastrin is a hormone secreted to stimulate the production of hydrochloric acid in the stomach.[5] Removal of part of the stomach can impair the negative feedback loop, resulting in elevated serum gastrin levels. The hypergastrinemia results in excess acid loss, leading to hypokalemic hypochloremic metabolic alkalosis.[5] The increase in gastric acid secretion can also predispose these patients to ulcers in the bladder and stomach.

Jejunum

The jejunum, with a relatively low number of tight junctions, is the least desirable bowel segment for urologic reconstruction.[6] Due to its increased permeability, there is a much higher fluid and electrolyte loss that occurs when jejunum is in contact with the urinary tract. Consequently, individuals who undergo reconstruction using these segments are at a much higher risk of metabolic complications and electrolyte imbalance, most notably hyponatremia, hypochloremia, hyperkalemia, azotemia, and metabolic acidosis.[10] These derangements are a result of the increase in sodium and chloride secretion into the urine with reabsorption of hydrogen and potassium ions.[11] This results in dehydration because fluid follows the sodium and chloride. As a consequence of dehydration, the renin-angiotensin system is activated, which causes increased aldosterone levels. With the increase in aldosterone, the kidneys conserve sodium and excrete potassium into the urine, whereby it is then reabsorbed by the jejunum segment in exchange for sodium.[12] This further perpetuates the hyperkalemia and hyponatremia. With an increase in serum potassium, renal acid excretion is hindered, leading to acidosis.[9] This is referred to as jejunum conduit syndrome in its most severe form and can affect up to 25% of patients.[12] Factors affecting severity of this syndrome include concurrent illness, length of segment used, and location of segment, with longer and more proximal segments resulting in more severe imbalances.[13,14] Because of its high rate of complications, use of jejunum is limited to patients for whom other bowel segments are undesirable due to either radiation, previous surgeries, or bowel disorders.[12]

Ileum and Colon

Ileum and colon are the most common segments used in urologic reconstruction and pose similar risks for metabolic and electrolyte derangements. Although used in both conduits and bladder reconstruction, the latter typically has more issues owing to the increased amount of time urine spends in contact with the bowel segment. The most common consequence is hyperchloremic metabolic acidosis, which occurs in 15% to 50% of patients.[5,15] The wide variability in estimation is largely related to the lack of standardized definition of acidosis for this population but is most commonly accepted at a venous bicarbonate less than 21 mmol/L.[16] The acidosis primarily results from ammonium reabsorption by the ileum and colon.[5] As urinary pH increases, so does the ammonium reabsorption. Further compounding the issue is the increase in bicarbonate and sodium excretion in exchange for chloride and hydrogen, which furthers acidosis.[15]

These issues are most pronounced in patients with renal or hepatic issues. With impaired renal function, the body has decreased capability to compensate for metabolic changes. The hepatic system plays an important role in regulation because the bowel segment retains its native blood supply with the venous return draining directly into the portal circulation.[9] With normal hepatic function, the liver can adapt and process the increased ammonium absorbed by the bowel. However, with mildly impaired hepatic function, prolonged retention of urine, or infection with urea-splitting organism such as *Pseudomonas*, *Klebsiella*, or *Proteus*, the ability of the liver to process the ammonium load may be insufficient. In severe cases, this can result in ammoniagenic coma.[17]

Related electrolyte abnormalities can include hypokalemia, hypocalcemia, and rarely hypomagnesemia.[15] Hypokalemia can be attributed to both intestinal loss as well as renal wasting. Because the ileum has better ability to reabsorb potassium, this is more common when colon is used in reconstruction.[18] Hypokalemia can be further exacerbated with correction of acidosis, which worsens potassium depletion by causing potassium to shift to the intracellular space.[19] Therefore, with correction of acidosis, special attention should be paid to potassium because supplementation is often necessary.

Hypocalcemia may result from both renal wasting and loss from bone stores.[15] With chronic metabolic acidosis, carbonate is mobilized from bone as a buffer, which results in calcium being released. The reabsorption of calcium is impaired in the kidneys due to acidosis, resulting in hypocalcaemia.

COMPLICATIONS RELATED TO BOWEL RESECTION

Although much of the literature has focused on the consequences of bowel being interposed in the urinary tract, complications can result from the loss of bowel segment as well. The degree to which a patient suffers bowel dysfunction is directly correlated to length and type of segment used. These effects are most pronounced when ileum is used. If gastric or jejunum segments are used, patients are less likely to suffer complications related to the loss of the segment.

Ileum

The most commonly cited reason for decreased quality of life related to these surgeries is the diarrhea patients often experience.[20] This can be seen with ileum resection due to decrease in bile salt and fat absorption. Bile salts are normally reabsorbed by the terminal ileum. With the loss of ileum, large quantities of bile salts enter the colon, causing mucosal irritation and resulting in diarrhea.[15] The decrease in fat absorption with loss of small bowel can lead steatorrhea, furthering the effects of diarrhea.

Diarrhea can be further compounded if the ileocecal valve is incorporated in the diversion. With loss of the ileocecal valve, patients may experience bacterial overgrowth, which can further hinder bile salt and fat absorption. The ileocecal valve also controls small bowel transit time. Loss of this valve decreases transit time and predisposes the patient to diarrhea.[5] Because of these complications, some surgeons may attempt to reconstruct the ileocecal valve if it is used in urologic reconstruction.

Related to loss of bile salts, patients may also experience lipid abnormalities. Serum cholesterol decreases with increase in length of ileum that is removed and, consequently, triglycerides increase.[21] Several mechanisms may explain this. With loss of bile acid reabsorption, the liver increases channeling of cholesterol to convert to bile acids, lowering serum cholesterol levels.[5] Lipid absorption also decreases related to loss of bile acid absorption. Finally, as a treatment of diarrhea, Cholestyramine is often given, which decreases cholesterol but can increase serum triglyceride levels. Impaired absorption of the fat-soluble vitamins A, D, E, and K may also occur, related to lipid malabsorption and use of cholestyramine for diarrhea.[5]

Patients may also experience vitamin B12 deficiency after resection of ileum. This is related to loss of intrinsic factor, which is required for enteral absorption of B12.[5] Because the body usually has significant B12 stores in the liver, the deficiency is not often seen until years after initial resection. It is important to be aware of this potential consequence, due to serious consequences of B12 deficiency, including megaloblastic anemia and peripheral nerve paresthesias.[11]

Colon

Like ileum resection, loss of colon may cause diarrhea in some patients. This can happen when the remaining colon length is unable to absorb the water and alkaline intestinal contents.[11] In severe cases, this can lead to dehydration and acidosis. However, most patients tolerate colon resection with less dysfunction than those undergoing ileum resection, provided the ascending colon remains intact.[5]

RELATED METABOLIC COMPLICATIONS
Bone Density

Although controversial in its level of significance, there is some evidence that the chronic metabolic acidosis induced through use of bowel in the urinary tract can lead to decrease in bone mineral density. This is a particular concern when these procedures are done in children because their bones are still developing and, as a result, they are at a higher risk for bone-related complications. In adults, this can contribute to the development of osteoporosis without early identification and intervention. These consequences are in part related to how the body buffers chronic acidosis. Carbonate is released from the bones in exchange for hydrogen ions, causing a release of calcium into circulation.[22] The increased serum calcium is then cleared through the kidneys, further depleting calcium. The acidosis also activates osteoclasts contributing to the bone demineralization.[11] In addition, the body's ability to absorb vitamin D and, as a consequence, absorb calcium may be impaired if ileum is used in the reconstruction due to loss of bile acids and fat malabsorption.[5] The acidosis further worsens this because it impairs renal activation of vitamin D.[11] These effects are exacerbated by even mild renal impairment, which is not uncommon in these patients. It is important to note, however, that with correction of acidosis, bone remineralization can occur.[23] This emphasizes the importance of monitoring for acidosis and treating even mild cases to prevent demineralization from occurring. Currently, there are no recommendations with regard to frequency of bone density screening for this population.

Stones

Patients with neobladders, continent cutaneous diversions, and augmentations are at a higher risk for bladder stones. Multiple conditions can contribute to this. First, the increase in mucus production can provide a nidus for stone formation by binding calcium from the urine.[24] Second, the diversions do not function the same as native bladders and are prone to incomplete emptying. The urinary stasis produced by this allows solutes to precipitate out of the urine and form stones. These patients also have chronic colonization and/or recurrent infections that can predispose them to stone formation. Finally, if any staples or sutures are exposed, this can form a nidus for stones. All of these factors can predispose patients to bladder stones that seem to increase in frequency as time progresses.[24]

Due to metabolic changes related to use of bowel in reconstruction, these patients are also at a greater risk for nephrolithiasis. There are several mechanisms that increase this risk. First is the metabolic acidosis, which is buffered by carbonate release from the bone. As previously discussed, this results in an increase in serum calcium, which is then excreted through the kidneys, causing hypercalciuria, a known risk factor for calcium stones. If ileum is used, there is an increased risk of oxalate stones. Under normal circumstances, calcium in the gastrointestinal tract binds to oxalate. With loss of ileum, there is an increase in bile salts being excreted, which binds with calcium, thereby allowing oxalate to remain unbound.[11] This unbound oxalate is absorbed and filtered out through the kidneys, which increases the risk of calcium oxalate stones. In addition, the diarrhea and loss of water reabsorption patients may experience with loss of bowel can lead to dehydration. This allows for supersaturation of stone constituents to precipitate out in the urine, causing the formation of stones. Furthermore, the renal excretion of citrate, a known stone inhibitor, is decreased in acidosis. This increases the formation of multiple types of stones.[25] Finally, chronic colonization of the diversion with bacteria can lead to struvite and/or carbonate apatite stones.[15] Due to the confluence of these factors, patients are at a higher risk for multiple types of nephrolithiasis.

Drug Absorption

It is important to note, in patients with bowel incorporated into their urologic tract, drug absorption may be altered. This applies to drugs that are secreted unchanged into the urine that can then be reabsorbed by the intestinal segment.[16] Methotrexate, phenytoin, theophylline, lithium, aminoglycoside antibiotics, ciprofloxacin, and β-lactam antibiotics are all among those that need drug-level monitoring in patients who have undergone this type of reconstruction.[2,16,27] In patients undergoing cisplatin-based chemotherapy, it has been advised to place a catheter to allow for urine drainage to minimize possibility of reabsorption from the urine.[3] It is important that patients who have undergone urologic reconstruction with intestinal segments be monitored for toxicity when these susceptible drugs are administered.

SUMMARY

When the gastrointestinal tract is used in urologic reconstruction, metabolic and electrolyte derangements may result. These can be caused by abnormal solute absorption from the urine or from the loss of the function originally provided by the segment in the gastrointestinal tract. The type of bowel segment used and the total amount of surface area that is exposed greatly influences the type and severity of complications that are seen. These can be exacerbated by prolonged urine retention, infection, or impairments in renal or hepatic function. Due to the nonspecific nature of symptoms these patients may present with, it is important to be aware of the potential metabolic and electrolyte abnormalities that may occur and carefully evaluate patients who have undergone this type of urologic reconstruction.

REFERENCES

1. Snyder CC. A new therapeutic concept of the exstrophied bladder. Plast Reconstr Surg Transplant Bull 1958;22(1):1–10.
2. Krajewski W, Piszczek R, Krajewska M, et al. Urinary diversion metabolic complications - underestimated problem. Adv Clin Exp Med 2014;23(4):633–8.
3. Hansen MH, Hayn M, Murray P. The use of bowel in urologic reconstructive surgery. Surg Clin North Am 2016;96(3):567–82.

4. McDougal WS. Bladder reconstruction following cystectomy by uretero-ileo-colourethrostomy. J Urol 1986;135(4):698–701.

5. Mills RD, Studer UE. Metabolic consequences of continent urinary diversion. J Urol 1999;161(4):1057–66.

6. Stampfer DS, McDougal WS, McGovern FJ. Metabolic and nutritional complications. Urol Clin North Am 1997;24(4):715–22.

7. Sinaiko E. Artificial bladder from segment of stomach and study of effect of urine on gastric secretion. Surg Gynecol Obstet 1956;102(4):433–8.

8. Adams M, Mitchell M, Rink RC. Gastrocystoplasty: an alternative solution to the problem of urological reconstruction in the severely compromised patient. J Urol 1988;140(5 Pt 2):1152–6.

9. Tanrikut C, McDougal WS. Acid-base and electrolyte disorders after urinary diversion. World J Urol 2004;22(3):168–71.

10. Dahl, Douglas M, McDougal WS. Use of intestinal segments in urinary diversion. Campbell-Walsh Urology 2007;3:2534–78.

11. Vasdev N, Moon A, Thorpe AC. Metabolic complications of urinary intestinal diversion. Indian J Urol 2013;29(4):310–5.

12. Klein EA, Montie JE, Montague DK, et al. Jejunal conduit urinary diversion. J Urol 1986;135(2):244–6.

13. Stein R, Schröder A, Thüroff JW. Bladder augmentation and urinary diversion in patients with neurogenic bladder: non-surgical considerations. J Pediatr Urol 2012;8(2):145–52.

14. Bonnheim DC, Petrelli NJ, Sternberg A, et al. The pathophysiology of the jejunal conduit syndrome and its exacerbation by parenteral hyperalimentation. J Surg Oncol 1984;26(3):172–5.

15. Van der Aa F, Joniau S, Van Den Branden M, et al. Metabolic changes after urinary diversion. Adv Urol 2011;2011:764325.

16. Bakke A, Jensen KM, Jonsson O, et al. The rationale behind recommendations for follow-up after urinary diversion: an evidence-based approach. Scand J Urol Nephrol 2007;41(4):261–9.

17. McDermott WV Jr. Diversion of urine to the intestines as a factor in ammoniagenic coma. N Engl J Med 1957;256(10):460–2.

18. Koch M, McDougal W. Nicotinic acid: treatment for the hyperchloremic acidosis following urinary diversion through intestinal segments. J Urol 1985;134(1):162–4.

19. Koff SA. Mechanism of electrolyte imbalance following urointestinal anastomosis. Urology 1975;5(1):109–14.

20. Joniau S, Benijts J, Van Kampen M, et al. Clinical experience with the N-shaped ileal neobladder: assessment of complications, voiding patterns, and quality of life in our series of 58 patients. Eur Urol 2005;47(5):666–73.

21. Miettinen T. Relationship between faecal bile acids, absorption of fat and vitamin b12, and serum lipids in patients with ileal resections. Eur J Clin Invest 1971;1(6):452–60.

22. Bettice J, Gamble JL. Skeletal buffering of acute metabolic acidosis. Am J Physiol 1975;229(6):1618–24.

23. Siklos P, Davie M, Jung R, et al. Osteomalacia in ureterosigmoidostomy: healing by correction of the acidosis. Br J Urol 1980;52(1):61–2.

24. Gough DCS. Enterocystoplasty. BJU Int 2001;88(7):739–43.

25. Zuckerman JM, Assimos DG. Hypocitraturia: pathophysiology and medical management. Rev Urol 2009;11(3):134–44.

26. DuBose TD. Acidosis and alkalosis. In: Longo DL, Fauci AS, Kasper DL, et al, editors. Harrisons principles of internal medicine. 18th edition. New York: McGraw Hill; 2012. p. 363–73.
27. Ekman I, Mansson W, Nyberg L. Absorption of drugs from continent caecal reservoir for urine. BJU International 1989;64(4):412–6.
28. Hoffbrand AV. Megaloblastic anemias. In: Longo DL, Fauci AS, Kasper DL, et al, editors. Harrisons principles of internal medicine. 18th edition. New York: McGraw Hill; 2012. p. 865.
29. Morrison G. Serum chloride. In: Walker HK, Hall WD, Hurst JW, editors. Clinical methods: the history, physical, and laboratory examinations. 3rd edition. Boston: Butterworths; 1990. Available at: http://www.ncbi.nlm.nih.gov/books/NBK309/. Accessed July 12, 2016.

Microvascular Fluid Resuscitation in Circulatory Shock

Shannan K. Hamlin, PhD, RN, ACNP-BC, AGACNP-BC, CCRN, NE-BC[a],*,
Penelope Z. Strauss, PhD, MSN, CRNA[b], Hsin-Mei Chen, PhD, MBA[c],
LaDonna Christy, MSN, RN, CCRN[d]

KEYWORDS

• Microcirculation • Shock • Hemodynamic coherence • Fluid • Oxygen transport

KEY POINTS

• The macrocirculation is the conduit for blood flow, whereas the microcirculation is responsible for fine-tuning capillary blood flow to maintain whole-body homeostasis.
• Microcirculatory shock persists after optimization of systemic hemodynamic measures.
• A loss of hemodynamic coherence between the macrocirculation and microcirculation exists in circulatory shock.
• Microcirculatory-guided fluid therapy based on direct visualization of the microcirculation is feasible to prevent the adverse outcomes associated with too little or too much fluid volume administration during resuscitation.

INTRODUCTION

In circulatory shock, cardiovascular optimization using fluid volume replacement is a widely accepted paradigm regardless of the shock subtype (hypovolemic, cardiogenic, obstruction, distributive). As one of the most common life-threatening conditions in critically ill patients, circulatory shock is an acute failure of the cardiovascular system to deliver sufficient oxygen to meet tissue oxygen demands. The result is tissue hypoxia with cellular dysfunction, organ dysfunction, and activation of anaerobic metabolism cellular pathways.

Disclosure: The authors have nothing to disclose.
[a] Center for Professional Excellence, Institute for Academic Medicine, Houston Methodist, 6565 Fannin, MGJ 11-016, Houston, TX 77030, USA; [b] Independent Consultant, 6122 Queensloch Drive, Houston, TX 77096, USA; [c] Institute for Academic Medicine, Houston Methodist, 6565 Fannin, MGJ 11-018, Houston, TX 77030, USA; [d] Center for Professional Excellence, Houston Methodist Hospital, 6565 Fannin, MGJ 11-017, Houston, TX 77030, USA
* Corresponding author.
E-mail address: SHamlin@HoustonMethodist.org

Under physiologic conditions, a complex integrated oxygen transport network involving the lungs, heart, macrovasculature, and microvasculature efficiently move oxygenated blood from the environment to the tissues where oxygen is used for cellular metabolism and waste products are removed. Although the cardiovascular system circulates blood throughout the large arteries and veins (macrocirculation), the microcirculation is responsible for blood flow regulation and red blood cell (RBC) distribution throughout individual organs.[1] The microcirculation is essential to normal organ perfusion and functioning so it is now considered a distinct vital organ of the cardiovascular system,[2] which is remarkable considering that evidence of microcirculatory shock persists even after optimization of macrocirculatory hemodynamics.

Hypovolemia is a component in all subtypes of shock pathophysiology, making fluid resuscitation a cornerstone of therapy.[3] Typically titrated to macrovascular hemodynamic end points, the goal with fluid volume administration is to increase cardiac output (CO), thereby promoting adequate tissue perfusion and oxygenation. Conceptually, the basis for fluid administration is found at the level of the heart in the Frank-Starling law of cardiac performance; for a given increase in preload an increase in stroke volume and CO will result, thereby augmenting global forward blood flow. This macrocirculatory view assumes an increase in global blood flow parallels an increase in microcirculatory blood flow with improvements in cellular oxygenation. However, evidence now shows microcirculatory independence from macrovascular fluid administration in circulatory shock and especially in septic shock. This article discusses current understanding of changes in microvascular perfusion and oxygenation under hypovolemic conditions associated with circulatory shock, and insights into microcirculatory-guided fluid therapy.

Physiologic Microcirculatory Oxygen Transport and Use

The cardiovascular system is an elaborate, highly integrated oxygen transport system with the salient purpose of delivering adequate amounts of oxygen to the tissues to meet cellular oxygen demands and remove metabolic waste products. The large arteries and veins of the macrocirculation are tightly controlled by vascular, neural, hormonal, and biochemical processes to ensure matched bulk oxygen-rich blood delivery to the tissues to meet metabolic demands.[4] Once oxygenated blood from the pulmonary system enters the left heart it is pumped to the large arteries of the macrocirculation. Blood is deoxygenated in the microvascular system to then reenter the macrocirculation and travel through the large veins to the right heart to repeat the process. See **Fig. 1**. Although the macrocirculation is the conduit for blood flow, the microcirculation executes the detailed purpose of the cardiovascular system, which is to oxygenate tissues and organs to maintain homeostasis.

The most distal part of the circulatory system is the microcirculation, which includes the arterioles, capillaries, and venules. These smaller vessels deliver and distribute oxygen and nutrients to the tissues for metabolic use and then remove the metabolic waste. The first to receive blood from the macrocirculation are the arterioles. Because arterioles have a thick smooth muscle layer, they have the ability to constrict and dilate in order to precisely regulate blood flow to individual tissues and organs. The internal diameter of the arteriole is approximately 30 μm. Vessel diameter is important to note because it relates to blood flow velocity or rate.

The capillaries are the exchange vessels that receive oxygenated blood from the arterioles and distribute it to the tissues where it is needed. Oxygen is first chemically dissociated with the hemoglobin molecule and it then diffuses through the capillary wall to reach the cell. The cell organelle mitochondria then serve as energy factories

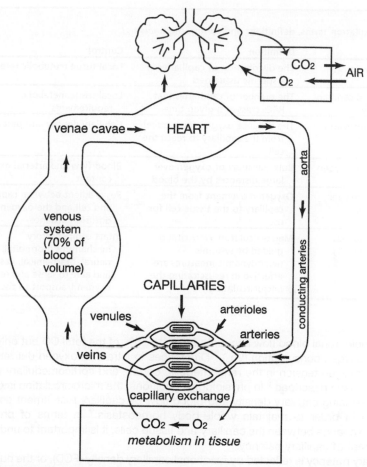

Fig. 1. The cardiovascular system. Oxygenated blood from the lungs enters the left heart from where it is pumped through the aorta, large arteries, and arterioles before entering the capillaries for gas exchange. Carbon dioxide (CO_2) and waste products diffuse from the tissues back to the capillaries, venules, and large veins to the right heart. (*From* Opie LH. Introductory cardiovascular concepts. The Heart Physiology, from Cell to Circulation. 3rd edition. Philadelphia: Lippincott-Raven; 1998. p. 3–15; with permission from Lionel Opie MD, lionel.opie@uct.ac.za.)

where oxygen is used to form energy through a cellular metabolic process called oxidative phosphorylation. Capillaries have an internal diameter of only 5 μm and, because they lack smooth muscle, they lack the ability to actively change their size.[5] Instead, capillaries are recruited (opened to blood flow) in times of increased oxygen demand, such with rigorous exercise, or capillaries can be derecruited (shutting down or limiting blood flow) when oxygen requirements are reduced. This physiologic capillary blood flow shunting permits timely precision of oxygenated blood flow during acute states of increased oxygen demand. In chronic hypoxic states (eg, pulmonary disease), capillaries adapt over time by increasing the distribution of capillaries, or capillary density.[6]

The capillary density is based on specific tissue metabolic demands and is known to vary (known as heterogeneity) both within and among organ tissue beds[4] (**Table 1**).

Table 1
Microcirculation terms, definitions and control mechanisms

Terms	Definition	Control
Capillary density	The distribution of capillaries in a specific tissue bed	Local tissue metabolic rate
Functional capillary density	The number of capillaries that RBCs cross at a given time	Local tissue metabolic requirements
Oxygen diffusion distance	The distance oxygen must travel from the capillary to reach the cell	Capillary density and patency
Convective oxygen transport	Bulk transport of oxygen over large distances by the blood	Blood flow and arterial oxygen content
Diffusive oxygen transport	Oxygen movement from the capillary to the tissue cell for use	Po_2 gradient between capillary and cell and the oxygen diffusion distance
Hemodynamic coherence	Macrocirculatory resuscitation guided by systemic hemodynamic measures are effective in resuscitating the microcirculatory	Intact compensatory mechanisms (hormonal, neural, biochemical, vascular) and able to sense and regulate oxygen transport to tissues

For example, renal blood flow accounts for up to 25% of the total CO but only 8% of the total oxygen consumption (Vo_2).[7] Differences in intrarenal oxygen delivery (Do_2), Vo_2, and oxygen tension in the renal medulla, cortex, and corticomedullary junction have also been described.[8] In physiologic conditions, the microcirculation is continuously fine-tuning capillary density and blood flow by capillary recruitment and derecruitment in order to maintain whole-body homeostasis.[9] In terms of promoting oxygen exchange between the capillary and tissue cells, it is important to understand the concept of capillary patency.

Capillary patency is reflected by functional capillary density (FCD), or the number of capillaries in a given area of tissue filled with actively flowing RBCs.[10] Direct visualization using hand-held microscopy is the gold standard for assessing capillary patency and therefore tissue perfusion.[4] An increase in FCD increases tissue oxygen tension (Po_2), allowing more oxygen availability to the tissues and reduces the oxygen diffusion distance, or the distance oxygen must travel to reach the mitochondria for use.[11] In summary, it is not enough to ensure adequate global Do_2; precise microvascular Do_2 within the organ according to tissue demand is needed.[12]

Convective and diffusive oxygen transport
Capillary blood flow and capillary density are critically important because they interact to determine tissue perfusion. To ensure the adequacy of oxygen to meet cellular oxygen demands, oxygen transport mechanisms must be functional and adaptive to changes in cellular oxygen needs. The bulk flow of oxygen-rich blood to the microcirculation, or convective oxygen transport, determines the overall oxygen available for tissue use. Convective oxygen transport depends on capillary blood flow (controlled upstream by the tone of arteriolar resistance vessels) and oxygen content.[13]

Oxygen is transported by diffusive oxygen transport from the capillary to the cell for use in cellular metabolism. Diffusive oxygen transport is determined by the differential partial pressure of oxygen (Po_2) gradient between the capillary and cell, and the oxygen diffusion distance.[14] When capillary density is reduced, this increases the oxygen diffusion distance, making it more difficult for oxygen to reach the mitochondria (**Fig. 2**). In low-flow states, the microcirculation is characterized by a decrease in capillary density with resulting increase in oxygen diffusion distance.[11] However, more important is the heterogeneous blood flow pattern, which means that adequately perfused capillaries can be in close proximity to nonperfused capillaries. It is therefore possible to have areas with hypoxic zones when the overall organ blood flow is adequate.[11]

MICROCIRCULATORY ALTERATIONS IN CIRCULATORY SHOCK

Circulatory shock is the most common life-threatening condition found in the intensive care unit (ICU).[3] Specifically, circulatory shock is characterized by hypoxia caused by inadequate cellular oxygen supply (abnormal convective oxygen transport), with or without dysoxia with impaired oxygen use (abnormal diffusive oxygen transport).[7] Although not necessarily exclusive, there are 4 primary pathophysiologic mechanisms that may result in shock: reduced intravascular volume (hypovolemic), cardiac pump failure (cardiogenic), obstruction of the circulation (obstructive), and distributive disorders of the peripheral circulation (distributive).[15] In a study with more than 1650 patients with shock in the ICU, septic shock (distributive) was the most common (62%) subtype of shock, followed by cardiogenic (16%) and hypovolemic (16%), with obstructive shock rarely occurring.[11] Note that, because of the inflammatory response as a consequence of persistent cellular hypoxia, all subtypes of shock may evolve into distributive shock.[13] Hypovolemic and cardiogenic shock are more easily characterized by a decrease in CO as a consequence of reduced intravascular volume and preload or a failing heart, both of which result in reduced macrocirculatory blood flow. In these types of shock, the adequacy of the microcirculation generally parallels that of the macrocirculation, a phenomenon termed hemodynamic coherence.[4]

Distributive or septic shock is more complex to characterize. Microcirculatory injury is a key development leading to multiple organ failure and death as the infectious insult adversely targets every aspect of microvascular blood flow and tissue oxygenation. Without timely reversal, the infectious insult will lead to a decrease in capillary density with resulting increased oxygen diffusion distance, maldistribution of blood flow, abnormal shunting of oxygenated blood, and impaired cellular oxygen use.[16] In this scenario, improved macrocirculatory parameters may not be paralleled in the microcirculation, creating a loss of hemodynamic coherence. Recent evidence also describes a significant loss of hemodynamic coherence as it relates to fluid volume resuscitation,[17–19] which is a cornerstone therapy in patients with septic shock.

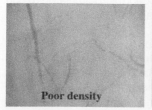
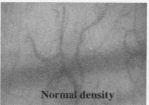
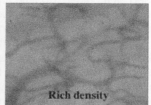

Poor density   Normal density   Rich density

Fig. 2. Different types of capillary density. (*From* Tanaka S, Harrois A, Nicolai C, et al. Qualitative real-time analysis by nurses of sublingual microcirculation in intensive care unit: the MICRONURSE study. Crit Care 2015;19:388.)

HEMODYNAMIC COHERENCE

Bedside monitoring of the microcirculation is currently beyond available technology. Macrocirculatory measures are more readily available so they continue to serve as microcirculatory indices despite a clear dissociation between global hemodynamics and microvascular perfusion.[11] Clinical surrogates used as global indicators of organ hypoperfusion include increased heart rate, hypotension, decreased urine output, increased lactic acid level, and acid-base abnormalities. The standard practice of using global hemodynamic and oxygen transport measures such as mean arterial pressure, CO, Do_2, Vo_2, and systemic vascular resistance as surrogates for measuring the microcirculation is based on the assumption that microcirculation perfusion is coupled with the macrocirculation.[20]

Hemodynamic coherence describes the long-standing premise that resuscitation designed to correct systemic hemodynamics will be effective in resuscitating the microcirculation. However, this is mistaken.[4] Numerous studies[21–24] have shown a loss of hemodynamic coherence between the macrocirculation and microcirculation in all subtypes of circulatory shock, with the most consistent findings in septic shock. Patients with persistent sublingual heterogeneous microcirculatory alterations irrespective of global hemodynamics have been shown to have a higher morbidity and mortality.[25,26] Loss of hemodynamic coherence likely explains the negative results from earlier studies that targeted normalization or supranormalization of hemodynamic and Do_2 variables.[27,28] The ability to assess in real time the state of the microcirculation during fluid resuscitation could lead to improved algorithms designed to resuscitate the microcirculation.

Tanaka and colleagues[29] evaluated real-time microcirculatory measures performed by ICU nurses using an incident dark-field illumination device (Cytocam-IDF) compared with the classic delayed semiquantitative analysis made by a physician. The results showed that bedside sublingual measurements performed by nurses were highly sensitive and specific for detecting impaired microvascular blood flow and reduced capillary density, and were comparable with the delayed semiquantitative analysis performed by physicians. These findings suggest that a real-time bedside technique for evaluating the microcirculation as part of standard nursing care is feasible, warranting further investigation.

MICROCIRCULATORY-GUIDED FLUID THERAPY

Optimal fluid volume occurs when FCD indicates optimal filling with the free flow of RBCs.[30] Improving microcirculatory perfusion and tissue oxygenation is the single most important goal when administering fluids in circulatory shock. However, managing fluid administration when considering the potential negative impact on the microcirculation is extremely complex, especially when global hemodynamic indices are used as a guide. Too little fluid volume can result in reduced microcirculatory blood flow, whereas too much volume can have a hemodilutional effect, thereby increasing the capillary diffusion distance.[30]

Common practice using the macrocirculatory approach is based on the Frank-Starling law of cardiac performance. Using this approach, clinicians base their fluid administration decisions on the notion that a positive relationship between preload and stroke volume exists; by increasing preload, stroke volume, CO, and perfusion pressure will increase.[3] However true it may be for the macrocirculation, the Frank-Starling law does not hold true for the microcirculation.

Four types of microcirculatory alterations have been found underlying the loss of hemodynamic coherence in circulatory shock states. These microcirculatory alterations can occur individually or in combination depending on the resuscitation modalities.[4] This classification system has been confirmed through direct visualization in various organ tissue beds.[31] Type 1 abnormalities relate to the heterogeneity in microcirculatory perfusion such that obstructed capillaries are in close proximity to functional capillaries. Type 1 alterations have commonly been shown in patients with infectious insults such as sepsis and are associated with significant adverse outcomes.[32] Interventions designed to correct type 1 alterations include both antiinflammatory and antibacterial agents to stabilize and protect the microcirculation and vasodilators to promote capillary patency.[4]

Type 2 alterations involve capillary hemodilution with loss of RBC-filled capillaries, thereby increasing the oxygen diffusion distance. This type of abnormality has been described in iatrogenic incidents, predominantly in cardiac surgery in which hemodilution was caused by excessive fluid administration.[33] Hemodilutional loss of coherence can be corrected with blood administration and monitored by maintaining an adequate hematocrit.[34] However, it stands to reason that overzealous fluid administration in all subtypes of circulatory shock could produce the same adverse effect on the microcirculation.

Type 3 microcirculatory abnormalities involve arterial vasoconstriction resulting in microcirculatory ischemia or increased venous pressures inducing microcirculatory tamponade, which results in reduced tissue oxygenation.[4] Type 3 loss of coherence results from unintended manipulation of systemic hemodynamic variables (ie, vasopressors) with resulting obstructed microcirculatory blood flow. Guidelines for the management of septic shock recommend fluid resuscitation in accordance with an increase in venous pressure.[35] However, venous pressures of 12 mm Hg or higher are associated with a significant reduction in microcirculatory perfusion caused by outflow obstruction.[36]

Type 4 abnormalities are associated with tissue edema, commonly found in sepsis or septic shock secondary to capillary leakage. Tissue edema results in increased oxygen diffusion distances between the capillary RBC and the tissue cell.[4] Often systemic hemodynamic variables indicate hypovolemia, particularly in septic shock, which invites further fluid administration causing further tissue edema and hypoxic insult.

From the aforementioned discussion it is evident that fluid administration designed to optimize intravascular filling is complex because both underfilling and overload can have adverse consequences on the microcirculation. The importance of considering the microcirculation when treating critically ill patients, especially those with circulatory shock, can no longer be ignored. It should be emphasized that, during resuscitation, the total fluid volume administered in circulatory shock is a formidable determinant of outcome.[37] However, microcirculatory research has investigated many therapeutic interventions, with microcirculatory-guided fluid administration indicating the greatest promise and readiness for implementation.[4]

SUMMARY

As Philippus von Hohenheim (1493–1541) stated so eloquently, "All things are poison, and nothing is without poison; only the dose permits something not to be poisonous."

The ultimate goal of fluid volume resuscitation in circulatory shock is to restore tissue perfusion and oxygenation. However, fluid therapy and monitoring guided by a Frank-Starling perspective using macrocirculatory end points may be harmful to the microcirculation in terms of impairment in connective and diffusive oxygen transport mechanisms. A loss of hemodynamic coherence between the macrocirculation and microcirculation should give clinicians pause when administering fluids if guidance is based on the assumption that macrocirculatory blood flow parallels microcirculation. The gold standard for guidance of fluid volume resuscitation should be based on optimization of the macrocirculation using systemic hemodynamic parameters and microcirculatory indices using direct visualization techniques. Future investigations should explore nurse-driven assessment of the microcirculation as part of ICU nursing standard monitoring and assessment.

REFERENCES

1. Hamlin SK, Parmley CL, Hanneman SK. Microcirculatory oxygen transport and utilization. Crit Care Nurs Clin North Am 2014;26(3):311–24.
2. Szopinski J, Kusza K, Semionow M. Microcirculatory responses to hypovolemic shock. J Trauma 2011;71(6):1779–88.
3. Gruartmoner G, Mesquida J, Ince C. Fluid therapy and the hypovolemic microcirculation. Curr Opin Crit Care 2015;21(4):276–84.
4. Ince C. Hemodynamic coherence and the rationale for monitoring the microcirculation. Crit Care 2015;19(Suppl 3):S8.
5. Mohrman DE, Heller LJ. Cardiovascular physiology. 7th edition. New York: McGraw-Hill Medical; 2010.
6. Saldivar E, Cabrales P, Tsai AG, et al. Microcirculatory changes during chronic adaptation to hypoxia. Am J Physiol Heart Circ Physiol 2003;285(5):H2064–71.
7. Ekbal NJ, Dyson A, Black C, et al. Monitoring tissue perfusion, oxygenation, and metabolism in critically ill patients. Chest 2013;143(6):1799–808.
8. Whitehouse T, Stotz M, Taylor V, et al. Tissue oxygen and hemodynamics in renal medulla, cortex, and corticomedullary junction during hemorrhage-reperfusion. Am J Physiol Renal Physiol 2006;291(3):F647–53.
9. De Backer D, Donadello K, Taccone FS, et al. Microcirculatory alterations: potential mechanisms and implications for therapy. Ann Intensive Care 2011;1(1):27.
10. den Uil CA, Klijn E, Lagrand WK, et al. The microcirculation in health and critical disease. Prog Cardiovasc Dis 2008;51(2):161–70.
11. De Backer D, Ortiz JA, Salgado D. Coupling microcirculation to systemic hemodynamics. Curr Opin Crit Care 2010;16(3):250–4.
12. Ellis CG, Jagger J, Sharpe M. The microcirculation as a functional system. Crit Care 2005;9(Suppl 4):S3–8.
13. Kanoore Edul VS, Ince C, Dubin A. What is microcirculatory shock? Curr Opin Crit Care 2015;21(3):245–52.
14. Bateman RM, Sharpe MD, Ellis CG. Bench-to-bedside review: microvascular dysfunction in sepsis–hemodynamics, oxygen transport, and nitric oxide. Crit Care 2003;7(5):359–73.
15. Weil MH, Shubin H. Proposed reclassification of shock states with special reference to distributive defects. Adv Exp Med Biol 1971;23(0):13–23.
16. Hamlin SK, Parmley CL, Hanneman SK. Microcirculatory alterations in shock states. Crit Care Nurs Clin North Am 2014;26(3):399–412.
17. Pottecher J, Deruddre S, Teboul JL, et al. Both passive leg raising and intravascular volume expansion improve sublingual microcirculatory perfusion in severe sepsis and septic shock patients. Intensive Care Med 2010;36(11):1867–74.

18. Ospina-Tascon G, Neves AP, Occhipinti G, et al. Effects of fluids on microvascular perfusion in patients with severe sepsis. Intensive Care Med 2010;36(6): 949–55.

19. Pranskunas A, Koopmans M, Koetsier PM, et al. Microcirculatory blood flow as a tool to select ICU patients eligible for fluid therapy. Intensive Care Med 2013; 39(4):612–9.

20. Benedik PS. Monitoring tissue blood flow and oxygenation: a brief review of emerging techniques. Crit Care Nurs Clin North Am 2014;26(3):345–56.

21. De Backer D, Creteur J, Dubois MJ, et al. The effects of dobutamine on microcirculatory alterations in patients with septic shock are independent of its systemic effects. Crit Care Med 2006;34(2):403–8.

22. Dubin A, Pozo MO, Casabella CA, et al. Increasing arterial blood pressure with norepinephrine does not improve microcirculatory blood flow: a prospective study. Crit Care 2009;13(3):R92.

23. Jhanji S, Stirling S, Patel N, et al. The effect of increasing doses of norepinephrine on tissue oxygenation and microvascular flow in patients with septic shock. Crit Care Med 2009;37(6):1961–6.

24. Ince C, Mik EG. Microcirculatory and mitochondrial hypoxia in sepsis, shock, and resuscitation. J Appl Physiol (1985) 2016;120(2):226–35.

25. Trzeciak S, McCoy JV, Phillip Dellinger R, et al. Early increases in microcirculatory perfusion during protocol-directed resuscitation are associated with reduced multi-organ failure at 24 h in patients with sepsis. Intensive Care Med 2008; 34(12):2210–7.

26. De Backer D, Donadello K, Sakr Y, et al. Microcirculatory alterations in patients with severe sepsis: impact of time of assessment and relationship with outcome. Crit Care Med 2013;41(3):791–9.

27. Gattinoni L, Brazzi L, Pelosi P, et al. A trial of goal-oriented hemodynamic therapy in critically ill patients. SvO2 Collaborative Group. N Engl J Med 1995;333(16): 1025–32.

28. Hayes MA, Timmins AC, Yau EH, et al. Elevation of systemic oxygen delivery in the treatment of critically ill patients. N Engl J Med 1994;330(24):1717–22.

29. Tanaka S, Harrois A, Nicolai C, et al. Qualitative real-time analysis by nurses of sublingual microcirculation in intensive care unit: the MICRONURSE study. Crit Care 2015;19:388.

30. Ince C. The rationale for microcirculatory guided fluid therapy. Curr Opin Crit Care 2014;20(3):301–8.

31. Elbers PW, Ince C. Mechanisms of critical illness—classifying microcirculatory flow abnormalities in distributive shock. Crit Care 2006;10(4):221.

32. Edul VS, Enrico C, Laviolle B, et al. Quantitative assessment of the microcirculation in healthy volunteers and in patients with septic shock. Crit Care Med 2012; 40(5):1443–8.

33. Atasever B, Boer C, Goedhart P, et al. Distinct alterations in sublingual microcirculatory blood flow and hemoglobin oxygenation in on-pump and off-pump coronary artery bypass graft surgery. J Cardiothorac Vasc Anesth 2011;25(5): 784–90.

34. Yuruk K, Almac E, Bezemer R, et al. Blood transfusions recruit the microcirculation during cardiac surgery. Transfusion 2011;51(5):961–7.

35. Dellinger RP, Levy MM, Carlet JM, et al. Surviving Sepsis Campaign: international guidelines for management of severe sepsis and septic shock: 2008. Crit Care Med 2008;36(1):296–327.

36. Vellinga NA, Ince C, Boerma EC. Elevated central venous pressure is associated with impairment of microcirculatory blood flow in sepsis: a hypothesis generating post hoc analysis. BMC Anesthesiol 2013;13:17.
37. Boyd JH, Forbes J, Nakada TA, et al. Fluid resuscitation in septic shock: a positive fluid balance and elevated central venous pressure are associated with increased mortality. Crit Care Med 2011;39(2):259–65.

Fluid Management in Lung Transplant Patients

Benjamin Stuart Schultze, PhD, MSN, MEd

KEYWORDS

- Lung transplant • Primary graft dysfunction • Pulmonary edema • Hypervolemia

KEY POINTS

- There are inconclusive data to guide the administration of fluids in lung transplant patients because rigorous randomized controlled trials have not been conducted.
- It seems that hypervolemia is associated with a disruption in the endothelial glycocalyx layer, which allows increased capillary permeability and edema.
- Thoracic surgery has been generally guided by the principle that hypervolemia is associated with negative outcomes and this same principle seems to apply to lung transplant patients.
- The role of both hypervolemia and hypovolemia in the development of primary graft dysfunction postoperatively is not yet known.

INTRODUCTION

Lung transplant is a lifesaving therapy for patients with end-stage pulmonary disease. According to the International Society for Heart and Lung Transplantation, each year in the United States, there are approximately 2000 lung transplants performed. At present, there are 11,000 lung transplant recipients alive in the United States.[1] The median survival for a bilateral lung transplant patient is 7 years, and 4.5 years for single lung transplants.[2] The leading cause of death for lung transplant patients occurs within the first 30 days posttransplant as a result of graft failure resulting in fulminant development of acute respiratory failure and diffuse alveolar damage. This condition occurs in approximately 25% of all lung transplants.[3] Furthermore, a form of acute lung injury that occurs in the first 72-hours post–lung transplant is known as primary graft dysfunction (PGD), which is not necessarily a harbinger of rejection. How fluid management and status in the first 30 days postoperatively affect lung transplants and the developments of PGD, early graft failure, and overall morbidity and mortality is poorly understood.

Disclosure: None.
Oregon Health & Science University, School of Nursing, Adult-Gerontlogy Acute Care Nurse Practitioner Program, 3455 S.W U.S. Veterans Hospital Road, Portland, OR 97239, USA
E-mail address: schultbe@ohsu.edu

Nurs Clin N Am 52 (2017) 301–308
http://dx.doi.org/10.1016/j.cnur.2017.01.007
0029-6465/17/© 2017 Elsevier Inc. All rights reserved.

Postoperative management of lung transplant patients consists of fluid and hemodynamic management, awakening from anesthesia, weaning from mechanical ventilator support, initiation of immunosuppression, infection prevention, and early detection of rejection.[4] However, the evidence to support a directional approach to fluid management in postoperative lung transplant patients is significantly lacking in terms of rigorous prospective randomized controlled trials. To date, the optimal fluid for volume replacement in postoperative lung transplant patients is unknown. Furthermore, there are no guidelines for the management of the early postoperative period following lung transplant.[5] In general, protocols seem to assist in recovery of thoracic patients.[6] This article addresses the complexities surrounding fluid management in lung transplant patients and offers evidence for an overall conservative approach to fluid resuscitation in the early postoperative period.

PRETRANSPLANT VARIABLES

Pulmonary edema in the transplanted lung patient is common.[7] There are multiple variables that likely influence the development of pulmonary edema in the postoperative phase following lung transplant (**Table 1**). To begin, it is important to understand how the condition of both the donor and the recipient before transplant potentially influences outcomes. Two of the primary variables that likely contribute to pulmonary edema in lung transplant patients and, potentially to survival, are the condition of the donor lung before transplant and the recipient patient's overall health status. Potential mechanisms of lung damage and edema before brain death include trauma; resuscitation; mechanical ventilation; aspiration of blood or gastric content; pneumonia; fluid management; and the inflammatory cascade of the individual, which is regulated by multiple cytokines.[8] The influence of inflammatory cytokines likely directly correlates with capillary permeability, resulting in pulmonary edema. Although the donor lung tissue is vulnerable to multiple insults compromising lung tissue, the recipients are also generally sick and are experiencing their own deterioration in health status, which likely influences edema development and outcomes in the postoperative period. The role of the transplants recipient's overall health and subsequent immunologic response with regard to a transplant is unknown. Several variables may influence a lung transplant outcome. One such variable is the main illness that results in the need for a transplant.

The 5 main illnesses that lead to lung transplant are idiopathic pulmonary fibrosis, chronic obstructive pulmonary disease, cystic fibrosis, idiopathic pulmonary arterial hypertension, and alpha1-antitrypsin deficiency emphysema. Each of these disease processes places significant stress on the body, resulting in significant deterioration over time in terms of functioning, muscle wasting, and susceptibility to infection and other illnesses. Each of the disease processes contributes to the body's inability to

Table 1
International Society for Heart and Lung Transplantation primary graft dysfunction definition and grading

Grade	Pao_2/Fio_2	Radiographic Infiltrates
0	>300	Absent
1	>300	Present
2	200–300	Present
3	<200	Present

mount a response to significant stressors. The stress of transplant is significant and it is likely that the body's pretransplant condition influences outcomes, specifically around fluid dynamics and edema development. A history of idiopathic pulmonary fibrosis, pulmonary arterial hypertension, significant smoking, and increased body mass index have been associated with worse outcomes and the development of PGD.[7,9]

The management of the donor patient before explantation of lungs is likely to directly influence the outcome of the transplant recipient.[10,11] One difficulty in determining how to manage potential lung donors is the heterogeneity of donors, their mechanism of injury resulting in death, and their overall health status before sustaining the injury resulting in death. It has been posited that the use of lung-protective ventilator strategies may protect against the development of atelectasis and neurogenic pulmonary edema within the lungs.[12] What this implies is that the posttransplant condition of both the donor and the recipient is likely to influence capillary permeability within the lung and this potentially complicates the use of fluids in the postoperative period.

Overall, the condition of both the donor and the recipient likely influences the overall response of the body to the stressors of the transplant.[12] The influence of these variables on the outcomes of lung transplant patients is not precisely known, which makes the development of postoperative guidelines difficult and means that postoperative lung transplant patients have multiple reactions to, and requirements for, volume management.

EXPLANTATION TO IMPLANTATION

During the removal of the donor lung, perfusion to the lung is stopped. Blood flow cessation results in ischemia and injury.[13] When blood flow is restored to the lung following implantation, the resulting injury that occurs from the return of blood flow is known as ischemia reperfusion and results in the development of PGD.[7,14] It is posited that the loss of mechanical force associated with blood flow and loss of oxygen delivery to the lung are the two main reasons for ischemic injury.[15] The complex physiology of lung transplant patients is also further complicated by the sympathetic burst and inflammation during brain death.[16] The secondary occurrence of inflammation is complex and beyond the scope of this article. However, the inflammatory cascade that results during cessation of blood flow primes the lungs for a cytokine response and is further exacerbated by the reintroduction of blood flow to the lungs during implantation. This process results in capillary leak secondary to cytokines and results in pulmonary edema. Increased cytokine levels in the pleural fluid of lung transplant recipients have been associated with acute rejection following transplant.[17] The Organ Care System, also known as "lung-in-the-box" technology is a potential avenue for reducing ischemic injury because it preserves both the circulation of blood and delivery of oxygen to occur while the lungs are external to the body and may reduce edema from the inflammatory cascade and subsequent capillary leak.

During surgery, the anesthesiology team is responsible for maintaining adequate perfusion pressure and cardiac circulation for adequate oxygen delivery to the body's tissues. Independent of thoracic surgery, all surgery induces an inflammatory and endocrine response that can affect the distribution of fluids throughout the body. The anesthesiology team is responsible for managing this initial response during surgery. Options for maintaining adequate pressure can be accomplished through the use of chemical inotropes and through the delivery of colloid and crystalloid fluids.

However, there are few studies that have examined the relationship between these modalities to maintain adequate circulation and outcomes in lung transplant recipients.[18] Many guidelines for restricting fluid administration during transplant exist, but the evidence behind this recommendation has not been precise.[19,20] In thoracic surgery patients in general, specifically those undergoing pneumonectomy, there has been an association between intraoperative fluid resuscitation in excess of 2000 mL as an independent risk factor in the development of postpneumonectomy pulmonary edema.[21] A recent study in dogs undergoing pneumonectomy indicated better outcomes in those with less fluid administered.[22] In short, it is not precisely known how intraoperative fluid management of lung transplant patients affects short-term and long-term outcomes; however, evidence now indicates that increased fluid resuscitation during surgery is associated with increased morbidity and mortality.

A recent retrospective cohort analysis of 494 patients showed that patients who received larger volumes of intraoperative fluid were associated with grade 3 PGD, which is the severest form of PGD ($P = .17$).[18] The International Society for Heart and Lung Transplantation considers a patient to have grade 3 PGD if the Pao$_2$/fraction of inspired oxygen (Fio$_2$) ratio is less than 200[23] (see **Table 1**). In addition, evidence has indicated that lung transplant patients receiving larger amounts of both crystalloid and colloid during surgery were associated with longer intensive care unit stays.[24] What the studies mentioned with regard to intraoperative fluid management and outcomes cannot answer is how the health of the person receiving the lungs affected the need for fluid resuscitation. A multivariate analysis of other factors was not conducted. It is possible that patients with more advanced forms of pulmonary disease requiring a transplant for survival may require greater amounts of fluid intraoperatively in order to maintain adequate perfusion pressure. In addition, patients requiring more fluids likely had a greater incidence of hemodynamic instability requiring fluid administration. If the patient was having increased hemodynamic instability from cytokine-mediated capillary leak, the resulting association between fluid administration and outcomes likely is not fully attributable to the amount or type of fluid the patient has received intraoperatively. Further studies are needed to stratify the health of transplant recipients and fluid requirements intraoperatively.

POSTOPERATIVE MANAGEMENT

Ideally, postoperative lung transplant patients would arrive at the intensive care unit and quickly move along a positive postoperative trajectory leading to early extubation, ambulation, and discharge to the ward. However, the reality is that many lung transplant patients experience postoperative complications. The early postoperative course seems to be associated with morbidity and mortality. In a recent retrospective analysis of 748 lung transplant patients, 92.78% experienced a postoperative complication.[25] As previously reviewed, the condition of the donor and recipient, and management in the operating room likely affects the postoperative trajectory. The question of how fluid management in the postoperative state affects both short-term and long-term outcomes is not fully elucidated. However, with such a high complication rate, future studies investigating the role of fluid in postoperative lung patients are warranted.

In general, thoracic surgery patients have been guided by the rule of minimizing fluid resuscitation when possible to reduce the chances of shifting fluids out of the vasculature space in response to the surgical instrumentation and secondary inflammation at the lung parenchyma. In thoracic surgery, there seems to be correlation between the extent of lung resection and intraoperatively administered amounts of fluid and the development of acute lung injury.[26] This correlation implies that the greater the extent of surgical involvement, the greater the inflammatory response that is likely attenuated by the use of fluid.[27] In lung transplant patients, the inflammatory response is already present in the individual undergoing donation. The lungs experience stress outside of the body and further stress during the transplant and subsequent adaptation to the recipient body.[28–30] Several inflammatory cells, cytokines, and chemokines have been implicated in the process resulting in edema development, which results in damage to the alveolar-capillary membrane.[31,32] This same process is present in non–lung transplant patients who develop acute lung injury and acute respiratory distress syndrome. This process can eventually lead to significant fibrosis and permanent impairment of the alveoli.[33,34] Previous experience with thoracic surgery patients likely dictates that a large inflammatory response will be present in lung transplant patients, making the effort of finding the right balance of volume resuscitation postoperatively more difficult.

A primary goal of post–lung transplant management is to avoid the development of acute lung injury that presents as PGD. However, the instrumentation and trauma that the lungs have experienced is likely to set the stage for issues with maintaining fluid status within the interstitium. One possibility for an increased propensity for fluid alterations is secondary to the trauma the lymphatic drainage system and the endothelial glycocalyx layer (EGL) of the lungs have experienced. The EGL is a network of glycoproteins and proteoglycans on endothelial cells.[35] Inflammatory mediators can impair a critical functions of the EGL, which is to keep fluid levels in equilibrium.[36,37] Alterations within the EGL cause and increase endothelial permeability, which likely results in the development of the pulmonary edema that has been seen in acute lung injury/PGD.[35] The basis for a conservative fluid resuscitation approach to managing thoracic surgery patients likely lies within the dysregulation of the EGL because hypervolemia can further impair the EGL that has already been altered through surgical instrumentation and the sequela of proinflammatory processes.[38,39] Possible ways to prevent injury to the EGL is not only to prevent hypervolemia but also to find appropriate interventions that may mitigate further damage to the EGL. Some possibilities for fluid resuscitation in post–thoracic surgery patients may be to use colloid infusions such as albumin instead.[40] However, the use of albumin has its own limitations and some clinicians think that albumin in postoperative lung transplant patients increases the sequestration of fluid within the pulmonary capillaries, further potentiating the effects of edema. Further studies examining this concept are needed. Nonetheless, postoperative lung transplant patients require fluid administration to thwart hemodynamic instability. This requirement leaves the care of post–lung transplant patients ambiguous and without rigorously developed protocols advising fluid administration postoperatively.

Postoperatively the goal is to maintain hemodynamic stability, but to allow the lungs to recover. This goal requires a balancing of volume status to ensure that hypovolemia does not occur and cause dysfunction of organs such as the kidneys, as well as avoiding hypervolemia resulting in tissue edema and organ dysfunction. Presently, there seems to a preponderance of evidence that volume resuscitation in lung transplant patients is detrimental to their recovery. Data suggesting that volume resuscitation in both thoracic and lung transplant patients is detrimental are lacking from rigorous randomized controlled trials.[27] As previously mentioned, the amount of volume given to thoracic surgery patients seems to correlate with pulmonary edema development, but the precise translation to lung transplant patients is unknown. However, without significant studies examining this correlation, a significant amount of data suggests that hypervolemia is detrimental. The extent of the damaging sequela of hypervolemia is unknown. Conservatively, finding the correct euvolemic state for each lung transplant patient is difficult because significant evidence to support arriving at this state of health are limited. Therefore, understanding the physiologic underpinnings of each lung transplant patient is important in delivering the optimal amount of fluid to promote optimal healing.

SUMMARY

Overall, there is a lack of randomized controlled trials examining the correlation between fluid volume delivery and outcomes in postoperative lung transplant patients. However, using thoracic surgery patients as a guide, the evidence suggests that hypervolemia correlates with pulmonary edema and should be avoided in lung transplant patients.[41] However, it is recognized that patients with hemodynamic instability may require volume for attenuation of this situation, but it can likely be mitigated with the use of inotropic medication to maintain adequate perfusion and avoid the development of edema.

REFERENCES

1. Tejwani V, Panchabhai TS, Kotloff RM, et al. Complications of lung transplantation: a roentgenographic perspective. Chest 2016;149(6):1535–45.
2. Stehlik J, Edwards LB, Kucheryavaya AY, et al. The registry of the International Society for Heart and Lung Transplantation: twenty-seventh official adult heart transplant report–2010. J Heart Lung Transplant 2010;29(10):1089–103.
3. Yusen RD, Edwards LB, Kucheryavaya AY, et al. The registry of the International Society for Heart and Lung Transplantation: thirty-second official adult lung and heart-lung transplantation report–2015; focus theme: early graft failure. J Heart Lung Transplant 2015;34(10):1264–77. Available at: http://www.jhltonline.org/article/S1053-2498(15)01389-3/abstract.
4. Leal S, Sacanell J, Riera J, et al. Early postoperative management of lung transplantation. Minerva Anestesiol 2014;80(11):1234–45. Available at: http://www.ncbi.nlm.nih.gov/entrez/query.fcgi?cmd=Retrieve&db=PubMed&dopt=Citation&list_uids=24518214.
5. Schuurmans MM, Benden C, Inci I. Practical approach to early postoperative management of lung transplant recipients. Swiss Med Wkly 2013;143:w13773.
6. French DG, Dilena M, LaPlante S, et al. Optimizing postoperative care protocols in thoracic surgery: best evidence and new technology. J Thorac Dis 2016; 8(Suppl 1):S3–11.
7. Diamond JM, Lee JC, Kawut SM, et al. Clinical risk factors for primary graft dysfunction after lung transplantation. Am J Respir Crit Care Med 2013;187(5):527–34. Available at: http://www.atsjournals.org/doi/full/10.1164/rccm.201210-1865OC.
8. Machuca TN, Cypel M, Yeung JC, et al. Protein expression profiling predicts graft performance in clinical ex vivo lung perfusion. Ann Surg 2015;261(3):591–7.
9. Samano MN, Fernandes LM, Baranauskas JC, et al. Risk factors and survival impact of primary graft dysfunction after lung transplantation in a single institution. Transplant Proc 2012;44(8):2462–8.
10. Hicks M, Hing A, Gao L, et al. Organ preservation. Methods Mol Biol 2006;333: 331–74.
11. Liu Y, Su L, Jiang SJ. Recipient-related clinical risk factors for primary graft dysfunction after lung transplantation: a systematic review and meta-analysis. PLoS One 2014;9(3):e92773.

12. Solidoro P, Schreiber A, Boffini M, et al. Improving donor lung suitability: from protective strategies to ex-vivo reconditioning. Minerva Med 2016;3(1):7–11. Available at: http://www.ncbi.nlm.nih.gov/entrez/query.fcgi?cmd=Retrieve&db=PubMed&dopt=Citation&list_uids=27308868.
13. van der Kaaij NP, Kluin J, Haitsma JJ, et al. Ischemia of the lung causes extensive long-term pulmonary injury: an experimental study. Respir Res 2008;9:28.
14. Porteous MK, Diamond JM, Christie JD. Primary graft dysfunction: lessons learned about the first 72 h after lung transplantation. Curr Opin Organ Transplant 2015;20(5):506–14.
15. Tao JQ, Sorokina EM, Vazquez Medina JP, et al. Onset of inflammation with ischemia: implications for donor lung preservation and transplant survival. Am J Transplant 2016;16(9):2598–611.
16. Weiss S, Kotsch K, Francuski M, et al. Brain death activates donor organs and is associated with a worse I/R injury after liver transplantation. Am J Transplant 2007;7(6):1584–93.
17. Camargo PC, Afonso Jr JE, Samano MN, et al. Cytokine levels in pleural fluid as markers of acute rejection after lung transplantation. J Bras Pneumol 2014;40(4):425–8.
18. Geube MA, Perez-Protto SE, McGrath TL, et al. Increased intraoperative fluid administration is associated with severe primary graft dysfunction after lung transplantation. Anesth Analg 2016;122(4):1081–8.
19. Shargall Y, Guenther G, Ahya VN, et al, ISHLT Working Group on Primary Lung Graft Dysfunction. Report of the ISHLT Working Group on Primary Lung Graft Dysfunction part VI: treatment. J Heart Lung Transplant 2005;24(10):1489–500.
20. Snell GI, Griffiths A, Levvey BJ, et al. Availability of lungs for transplantation: exploring the real potential of the donor pool. J Heart Lung Transplant 2008;27(6):662–7.
21. Zeldin RA, Normandin D, Landtwing D, et al. Postpneumonectomy pulmonary edema. J Thorac Cardiovasc Surg 1984;87(3):359–65. Available at: http://www.ncbi.nlm.nih.gov/entrez/query.fcgi?cmd=Retrieve&db=PubMed&dopt=Citation&list_uids=6700243.
22. Cruz RJ Jr, Tsutsui JM, Magno P, et al. Effects of fluid resuscitation on cardiovascular performance after posttraumatic pneumonectomy. J Trauma 2010;68(3):604–10. Available at: http://journals.lww.com/jtrauma/Abstract/2010/03000/Effects_of_Fluid_Resuscitation_on_Cardiovascular.19.aspx.
23. Oto T, Levvey BJ, Snell GI. Potential refinements of the International Society for Heart and Lung Transplantation primary graft dysfunction grading system. J Heart Lung Transplant 2007;26(5):431–6.
24. McIlroy DR, Pilcher DV, Snell GI. Does anaesthetic management affect early outcomes after lung transplant? An exploratory analysis. Br J Anaesth 2009;102(4):506–14.
25. Chan EG, Bianco V, Richards T, et al. The ripple effect of a complication in lung transplantation: evidence for increased long-term survival risk. J Thorac Cardiovasc Surg 2016;151(4):1171–9.
26. Licker M, Diaper J, Villiger Y, et al. Impact of intraoperative lung-protective interventions in patients undergoing lung cancer surgery. Crit Care 2009;13(2):R41.
27. Searl CP, Perrino A. Fluid management in thoracic surgery. Anesthesiol Clin 2012;30(4):641–55.
28. Altun GT, Arslantaş MK, Cinel İ. Primary graft dysfunction after lung transplantation. Turk J Anaesthesiol Reanim 2015;43(6):418–23.

29. Gohrbandt B, Simon AR, Warnecke G, et al. Lung preservation with Perfadex or Celsior in clinical transplantation: a retrospective single-center analysis of outcomes. Transplantation 2015;99(9):1933–9.
30. Schuurmans MM, Tini GM, Zuercher A, et al. Practical approach to emergencies in lung transplant recipients: how we do it. Respiration 2012;84(2):163–75.
31. Greenland JR, Xu X, Sayah DM, et al. Mast cells in a murine lung ischemia-reperfusion model of primary graft dysfunction. Respir Res 2014;15:95.
32. McClintock D, Zhuo H, Wickersham N, et al. Biomarkers of inflammation, coagulation and fibrinolysis predict mortality in acute lung injury. Crit Care 2008;12(2): R41.
33. Lee JW, Fang X, Dolganov G, et al. Acute lung injury edema fluid decreases net fluid transport across human alveolar epithelial type II cells. J Biol Chem 2007; 282(33):24109–19.
34. Olman MA, White KE, Ware LB, et al. Pulmonary edema fluid from patients with early lung injury stimulates fibroblast proliferation through IL-1 beta-induced IL-6 expression. J Immunol 2004;172(4):2668–77. Available at: http://www.ncbi. nlm.nih.gov/entrez/query.fcgi?cmd=Retrieve&db=PubMed&dopt=Citation&list_ uids=14764742.
35. Chau EH, Slinger P. Perioperative fluid management for pulmonary resection surgery and esophagectomy. Semin Cardiothorac Vasc Anesth 2014;18(1):36–44.
36. Wang L, Huang X, Kong G, et al. Ulinastatin attenuates pulmonary endothelial glycocalyx damage and inhibits endothelial heparanase activity in LPS-induced ARDS. Biochem Biophys Res Commun 2016;478(2):669–75.
37. Yang Y, Schmidt EP. The endothelial glycocalyx: an important regulator of the pulmonary vascular barrier. Tissue Barriers 2013;1(1). http://dx.doi.org/10.4161/tisb. 23494.
38. Bruegger D, Jacob M, Rehm M, et al. Atrial natriuretic peptide induces shedding of endothelial glycocalyx in coronary vascular bed of guinea pig hearts. Am J Physiol Heart Circ Physiol 2005;289(5):H1993–9.
39. Chappell D, Bruegger D, Potzel J, et al. Hypervolemia increases release of atrial natriuretic peptide and shedding of the endothelial glycocalyx. Crit Care 2014; 18(5):538.
40. Jacob M, Paul O, Mehringer L, et al. Albumin augmentation improves condition of guinea pig hearts after 4 hr of cold ischemia. Transplantation 2009;87(7):956–65.
41. Assaad S, Popescu W, Perrino A. Fluid management in thoracic surgery. Curr Opin Anaesthesiol 2013;26(1):31–9.

Tumor Lysis Syndrome
A Unique Solute Disturbance

Penelope Z. Strauss, PhD, MSN, CRNA[a],*,
Shannan K. Hamlin, PhD, RN, ACNP-BC, AGACNP-BC, CCRN, NE-BC[b], Johnny Dang, DNP, CRNA[c]

KEYWORDS

- Tumor lysis syndrome • Hyperuricemia • Hyperphosphatemia • Hyperkalemia
- Malignant cell metabolism

KEY POINTS

- Any patient with a cancer diagnosis who presents with electrolyte disorders or acute renal insufficiency should be evaluated for tumor lysis syndrome.
- Patients with tumor lysis syndrome may present with hyperuricemia, hyperphosphatemia, hypocalcemia, and/or hyperkalemia.
- Tumor lysis syndrome is highly associated with hematologic or bulky tumors, but may also occur in other types of cancer.
- Rasburicase reduces existing uric acid levels; allopurinol only prevents the formation of uric acid.
- Rasburicase is contraindicated to patients with glucose-6-phosphate dehydrogenase deficiency, therefore patients of African and Mediterranean descent should be screened before treatment.

Tumor lysis syndrome (TLS) is a worst-case scenario of specific electrolyte disturbances in which a sudden destruction of cancer cells releases massive amounts of intracellular solute into the general circulation. The abrupt increases in the levels of extracellular uric acid, phosphate, and potassium threaten cardiac and renal function, along with precipitating significant hypocalcemia that elicits central nervous system symptoms.[1,2] When the mass effects of solute overwhelm the body's ability for excretion, the patient may develop potentially fatal cardiac dysrhythmias or acute renal failure. Although historically associated with the initiation of chemotherapy in hematologic malignancy, TLS is now known to occur in the absence of exposure to

[a] Independent Consultant, 6122 Queensloch Drive, Houston, TX 77096, USA; [b] Center for Professional Excellence, Institute for Academic Medicine, Houston Methodist Hospital, 6565 Fannin, MGJ 11-017, Houston, TX 77030, USA; [c] Department of Acute and Continuing Care, University of Texas Health Science Center at Houston, 6901 Bertner Avenue SON 654, Houston, TX 77030, USA
* Corresponding author.
E-mail address: psvillars@gmail.com

Nurs Clin N Am 52 (2017) 309–320
http://dx.doi.org/10.1016/j.cnur.2017.01.008
0029-6465/17/© 2017 Elsevier Inc. All rights reserved.

nursing.theclinics.com

chemotherapy or radiotherapy (spontaneous TLS), and in a variety of solid tumors if treated with powerful cytotoxic agents.[3] A high index of suspicion has now become warranted in patients with many types of cancer because preventive measures and early recognition increase the opportunity for successful medical treatment of this oncologic emergency. The high acuity of both affected and at-risk patients suggests that the critical care team should not only be well versed in the causes and management of this disorder, but should be involved early in the course of their clinical care.[4]

PATHOPHYSIOLOGY OF TUMOR LYSIS SYNDROME

Cancers cells reproduce quickly and, when combined with a high malignant cell burden or in bulky tumors, these cells are a rich source of intracellular electrolytes and organic substances. Lysis of cancer cells releases typically compartmentalized nucleic acids, intracellular proteins, and electrolytes into the circulation, often overwhelming the compensatory mechanisms of homeostasis.[2] Although slow or subtle increases in uric acid, phosphate, or potassium may be tolerated, rapid and dramatic increases in plasma levels can become life threatening. In the presence of preexisting renal dysfunction or increased baseline levels of these solutes, rapid solute accumulation increases the risk of TLS.

Hyperuricemia and Acute Uric Acid Nephropathy

Unlike hemolysis of anucleated red blood cells, the lysis of tumor cells releases large amounts of nuclear material, including the building blocks deoxyribonucleic and ribonucleic acid (DNA and RNA). This release introduces free purines (adenine and guanosine), pyrimidines (cytosine, thymine, and uracil), and phosphate into the plasma. Although the nitrogen in pyrimidines is excreted in the form of water-soluble urea, purine metabolism leads to the production of uric acid. Functioning kidneys can effectively excrete excess urea, but the excretion of largely insoluble uric acid is transport dependent, and thus more problematic in the context of extremely high tubular loads. Urate is both reabsorbed and secreted in the proximal tubule, and the balance of these processes determines the eventual plasma level.[5,6]

When a high load of urate in acidic tubular fluid arrives in the distal tubule and collecting ducts, the mostly unionized uric acid precipitates. In TLS, monosodium urate crystal formation can obstruct renal tubules and cause renal injury, particularly in the presence of dehydration. Uric acid may also be directly nephrotoxic by several mechanisms.[7] First, uric acid inactivates the endogenous vasodilator nitric oxide, contributing to renal vasoconstriction and ischemia. Second, vascular smooth muscle exposed to uric acid produces proinflammatory mediators that can cause tissue injury. Third, uric acid can inhibit proliferation of cells in the proximal tubule which comprises the primary route of electrolyte handling in the kidney. Thus, an increasing serum uric acid level is associated with a progressively increased risk of TLS and acute kidney injury.[8]

Hyperphosphatemia and Secondary Hypocalcemia

Intracellular fluid has a high concentration of inorganic phosphate and, along with the phosphate backbones of DNA and RNA, spillage of cell contents can cause significant hyperphosphatemia. Rapidly proliferating malignant cells are said to contain higher levels of phosphate than normal cells, which significantly augments the plasma phosphate load after cell lysis.[9,10] These conclusions were inferred from analysis of white cell counts and plasma phosphorous levels before and after initiation of chemotherapy and tumor lysis in patients with lymphoma and leukemia.[10] As leukocyte counts decrease, serum and urinary phosphate levels increase sharply. Normally functioning kidneys can excrete excess phosphate; however, high phosphate levels trigger chelation with calcium. The precipitation of calcium phosphate crystals in soft tissues and renal tubules causes a secondary hypocalcemia. The formation of both uric acid crystals and calcium phosphate crystals in the renal tubules can cause an obstructive nephropathy. Along with the development of a decreased glomerular filtration rate, hyperphosphatemia is worsened as acute renal injury reduces the ability to excrete phosphate. As renal failure ensues, fluid retention can elicit pulmonary edema.

As noted, hypocalcemia is a direct result of the hyperphosphatemia because these electrolytes have a reciprocal relationship. Acute change in ionized calcium causes muscular hyperexcitability that elicits laryngeal stridor, dysphagia, and bronchospasm, along with paresthesias, tetany, or seizures. Prolonged QT syndrome, syncope, and cardiac failure can all occur because of hypocalcemia.[11]

Hyperkalemia and Cardiac Dysrhythmias

Hyperkalemia is often the first electrolyte disorder to manifest in TLS.[12] High intracellular potassium concentrations lead to hyperkalemia in any situation of rapid cell lysis, including massive tissue or crush injury (rhabdomyolysis), malignant hyperthermia, rapid infusion of erythrocytes, and TLS. Life-threatening manifestations of hyperkalemia occur in both the neuromuscular (weakness, cramps, paresthesia, or paralysis) and cardiac (dysrhythmias, ventricular tachycardia or fibrillation, syncope, or sudden death) systems.[13] The occurrence of simultaneous hyperkalemia and hypocalcemia is not well documented outside of tumor lysis scenarios. In one case report, despite receiving the recommended preventive strategies, a patient with intermediate-grade non-Hodgkin lymphoma had an irreversible asystolic event after chemotherapy initiation.[14] Thirty minutes before the arrest, the documented potassium level was 7.8 mmol/L and calcium level was 1.79 mmol/L. Although calcium gluconate was administered as part of the hyperkalemia treatment, the presence of relative hypocalcemia was potentially a contributory factor. This finding suggests that doses of more bioavailable calcium (calcium chloride rather than calcium gluconate) may be warranted when resuscitating patients with TLS in extremis.

DEFINING TUMOR LYSIS SYNDROME

Standard definitions of TLS are based on the patient's condition at presentation and are classed as laboratory TLS or clinical TLS, as shown in **Table 1**.[13] The diagnosis of laboratory TLS requires a current evaluation of uric acid, potassium, phosphate, or calcium levels in otherwise asymptomatic or mildly symptomatic patients. Criteria for laboratory TLS may be based on absolute solute values, or relative values compared with patient baseline. In addition, these abnormal values must develop within 3 days before, or up to 7 days after, the initiation of chemotherapy.[13] Symptomatic TLS assumes that laboratory values are abnormal because the patients present with acute renal insufficiency, significant cardiac dysrhythmias, seizures, or sudden death.

TRACKING RISK FOR TUMOR LYSIS SYNDROME

At-risk patients for TLS are well defined and are listed in **Table 2**. The syndrome may also present in patients with cancer who are considered low risk, following the initiation of chemotherapy, or spontaneously. In hematologic cancers, the cancer cell burden provides an indication of relative risk because the destruction of a large number of cells is more likely to elicit TLS.

Table 1
Cairo and Bishop[13] definitions of tumor lysis syndrome

Laboratory TLS[a]	
Uric acid	$\geq$476 μmol/L or 25% increase from baseline
Potassium	$\geq$6.0 mmol/L or 25% increase from baseline
Phosphorous	$\geq$2.1 mmol/L children, $\geq$1.45 mmol/L adults, or 25% increase from baseline
Calcium	$\leq$1.75 mmol/L or 25% decrease from baseline
Clinical TLS = Laboratory TLS and 1 or more of:	
Creatinine level $\geq$1.5 times upper limit of normal for age and sex	
Cardiac arrhythmia or sudden death[b]	
Seizure[b]	

[a] Laboratory TLS defined as any 2 or more values that meet criteria and occur within 3 days before or 7 days after chemotherapy initiation, in the presence of adequate hydration and treatment with a hypouricemic agent.
[b] Not attributable to a therapeutic agent or other identifiable cause.
From Cairo MS, Bishop M. Tumour lysis syndrome: new therapeutic strategies and classification. Br J Haematol 2004;127(1):3–11; with permission.

In addition, cancer cells undergo a metabolic reprogramming and show a very high metabolic rate characterized by increased glycolytic activity. This common feature of cancer cells is typified by abnormal glucose metabolism via an *aerobic* glycolysis. That is, glucose consumption occurs via glycolysis despite the availability of oxygen; this is termed the Warburg effect. Most energy production in cancer cells results from the conversion of pyruvate to lactate instead of pyruvate progressing into the mitochondrial citric acid cycle and oxidative phosphorylation.[15]

This metabolic phenomenon is evidenced by the upregulation and increased concentration of lactate dehydrogenase (LDH), the key enzyme in the final step of the glycolytic conversion of pyruvate to lactate.[16] Of the known LDH isoforms, LDH-5 or LDH-A is primarily expressed in cancer cells.[17,18] Thus, high levels of LDH-A are considered a sign of a high tumor burden and may indicate the degree of tumor aggressiveness.[16,19] For this reason, levels of LDH are used to define the threshold between risk factor classes.

Upregulation of LDH occurs in some types of cancer and is generally associated with tumor angiogenesis.[16] Increases in vascular endothelial growth factor (VEGF) expression are correlated with LDH levels in gastric cancer, suggesting that LDH may be a useful prognostic measure for VEGF-targeted cancer therapy.[20] LDH has been suggested as a prognostic indicator of poor outcomes in a variety of hematologic cancers and breast cancer with bone metastasis.[17,18]

Additional risk factors for TLS are present for patients who may ingest drugs that increase uric acid levels or contribute to impaired renal function. Commonly used uricogenic drugs include alcohol, ascorbic acid, aspirin, caffeine, cisplatin, diazoxide, thiazide diuretics, ethambutol or pyrazinamide (antituberculosis agents), levodopa or methyldopa, nicotinic acid (niacin), phenothiazines, and theophylline.[12] It would be prudent to avoid other known renal vasoconstrictors, such as nonsteroidal antiinflammatory drugs and iodinated contrast agents, to reduce the risk of renal compromise.[7]

Cases of spontaneous TLS have been reported in a variety of circumstances, some of which are summarized in **Table 3**. In many cases, symptoms of tumor lysis were the

Table 2
Hematologic conditions associated with tumor lysis syndrome

Risk Category	Diagnosis	Contributing Risk Factor
Very high	Burkitt lymphoma stage III/IV	LDH >2× upper limit
	Acute lymphoblastic leukemia	WBC >100 × 10^9/L or
		LDH >2× upper limit
	Acute myeloid leukemia	WBC >100 × 10^9/L
Intermediate	Burkitt lymphoma	LDH <2× upper limit
	Adult intermediate-grade NHL	LDH >2× upper limit
	Lymphoblastic lymphoma stage III/IV	LDH >2× upper limit
	Childhood intermediate-grade NHL	
	Childhood anaplastic large cell lymphoma stage III/IV	
	Acute lymphoblastic leukemia	WBC <100 × 10^9/L or
		LDH<2× upper limit
	Acute myeloid leukemia	WBC 25–100 × 10^9/L or
		WBC <25 × 10^9/L and
		LDH >2× upper limit
	Chronic lymphocytic leukemia	If treated with fludarabine/ rituximab or
		WBC >50 × 10^9/L
	Chronic myeloid leukemia	If experiencing an accelerated blast crisis
Low	Indolent NHL	
	Adult anaplastic large cell lymphoma	
	Adult intermediate-grade NHL	LDH <2× upper limit
	Lymphoblastic lymphoma stage I/II	LDH <2× upper limit
	Hodgkin lymphoma (most patients)	
	Acute myeloid leukemia	WBC <25 × 10^9/L and LDH <2× upper limit
	Chronic lymphocytic leukemia (most patients)	
	Chronic myeloid leukemia (most patients)	
	Multiple myeloma (in the absence of other risk factors)	

Abbreviations: LDH, lactate dehydrogenase; NHL, non-Hodgkin lymphoma; WBC, white blood cell count.

Data from Will A, Tholouli E. The clinical management of tumour lysis syndrome in haematological malignancies. Br J Haematol 2011;154:3–13.

first indication that a malignancy existed. These patients may present to the emergency room or critical care unit at institutions not associated with their oncology care. Thus a thorough history and physical examination, and a high index of suspicion when a cancer diagnosis is elicited, can speed an appropriate diagnosis.

PREVENTION OF TUMOR LYSIS SYNDROME

Thoughtful risk stratification and consideration of patient comorbidities are key to preventing TLS. Moderate-risk and high-risk patients should receive rigorous fluid hydration and pharmacologic prophylaxis should be implemented before chemotherapy or radiotherapy. Formal assessment of fluid balance (input and output) should occur every 6 hours, and electrolyte testing should occur every 6 to 12 hours in high-risk to moderate-risk patients, respectively.[2] Recent guidelines on the management of TLS using the grading of recommendations, assessment, development and

Table 3
Examples of spontaneous tumor lysis syndrome

Year	Patient and Presentation	Diagnosis	Outcome	Possible Contributor
Daly et al,[21] 2016	5-y-old boy presented with gross hematuria, lethargy, and right-sided abdominal pain	Uric acid nephrolithiasis; T-cell acute lymphoblastic leukemia	Survived	
Shenoy et al,[22] 2015	6-mo-old infant presented with fever and loose, bloody stools for 15 d	Acute myeloid leukemia; acute renal failure	Died of septicemia	
Chubb et al,[23] 2010	32-y-old man presented with painful abdominal distension, constipation and vomiting	Small bowel lesion; Burkitt lymphoma	Survived	Succinylcholine for RSI; low-dose hydrocortisone infusion after surgery; intraoperative tumor manipulation
Sinha et al,[24] 2009	7-y-old boy with neuroectodermal tumor treated with chemotherapy and radiotherapy, brought to surgery for tumor debulking	Cardiovascular collapse after anesthesia induction; severe metabolic acidosis and symptoms of TLS unresponsive to treatment	Unknown (parents left against medical advice after >1 mo of peritoneal dialysis)	
McDonnell et al,[25] 2008	3-y-old boy presented for elective adenotonsillectomy	Postoperative respiratory failure and shock; B-cell acute lymphoblastic leukemia	POD 2 hypoxic encephalopathy; died on POD 3	Received single-dose dexamethasone (0.25 mg/kg as PONV prophylaxis)
Lee et al,[26] 2007	6-y-old boy presented with abdominal distension and dyspnea, massive bilateral pleural effusion	Burkitt lymphoma	Survived	Cardiovascular collapse during staging laparotomy
Duzova et al,[27] 2001	11-y-old boy presented with malaise and weight loss	Acute lymphoblastic leukemia; received single-dose prednisolone PO	Both patients survived	Both patients received prophylactic alkaline diuresis and allopurinol before chemotherapy
	13-y-old male presented with malaise, fever and loss of appetite	Acute lymphoblastic leukemia; received 2 doses methylprednisolone		

Abbreviations: PO, by mouth; POD, postoperative day; PONV, postoperative nausea and vomiting; RSI, rapid sequence induction.

evaluations (GRADE) system of evidence evaluation have been published, and show that many aspects of TLS management are empirical and have not been subject to testing with a high level of rigor.[12,28] Thus, the GRADE guidelines in **Table 4** for the prophylaxis of TLS represent the facets of prophylactic treatment for which consensus has been reached.

TUMOR LYSIS SYNDROME TREATMENT IS SOLUTE SPECIFIC

Treatment of TLS addresses its primary metabolic disturbances: hyperuricemia, hyperphosphatemia, hyperkalemia, and hypocalcemia. Treatment of laboratory abnormalities should be prioritized by treating life-threatening or potentially life-threatening issues first, followed by symptomatic electrolyte disorders. In general, asymptomatic electrolyte abnormalities should be monitored but not actively treated. GRADE-based guidelines for the treatment of TLS are shown in **Table 5**, and represent the facets of acute treatment for which consensus has been reached.[12,28]

Table 4
Guidelines for prophylaxis of tumor lysis syndrome

Grade of Recommendation	Recommendation
1B. Strongly recommended based on moderate-quality evidence	Any patient with a hematologic malignancy should receive a risk assessment for TLS High-risk patients should be offered prophylaxis with rasburicase as well as increased hydration Urate samples taken from patients on rasburicase must be sent on ice to prevent false low results
1C. Strongly recommended based on low-quality evidence	In patients on rasburicase, efforts to alkalinize urine are not recommended
2C. Weak recommendation based on low-quality evidence	Low-risk patients managed with careful monitoring of fluid status and solute concentrations; care team should have a low threshold for instituting increased hydration and allopurinol Intermediate-risk patients should be offered up to 7 d of allopurinol prophylaxis and increased hydration after chemotherapy initiation or until risk of TLS is resolved High-risk adults in the absence of laboratory or clinical TLS: preventive strategies include a single 3-mg dose of rasburicase followed by very close monitoring of hydration and solute concentrations; repeat dosing PRN High-risk children in the absence of laboratory or clinical TLS: preventive strategies include single 0.2 mg/kg dose of rasburicase followed by close monitoring for evidence of TLS If rasburicase is used, do not add allopurinol because it may decrease efficacy of rasburicase Rasburicase is contraindicated in patients with G6PD deficiency: treat with fluid and allopurinol only

Abbreviations: G6PD, glucose-6-phosphate dehydrogenase; PRN, as needed.
Adapted from Jones GL, Will A, Jackson GH, et al. Guidelines for the management of tumour lysis syndrome in adults and children with haematological malignancies on behalf of the British Committee for Standards in Haematology. Br J Haematol 2015;169(5):661–71; with permission.

Table 5
Guidelines for treatment of tumor lysis syndrome

Grade of Recommendation	Recommendation
1A. Strongly recommended based on high-quality evidence	Do not add potassium to the hydration fluids Intractable fluid overload, hyperkalemia, hyperuricemia, hyperphosphatemia, or hypocalcemia are indications for renal dialysis Dialysis should be continued until complete recovery of renal function, full resolution of electrolyte balance, and recovery of appropriate urine output
1B. Strongly recommended based on moderate-quality evidence	Unless contraindicated, patients with TLS should receive 0.2 mg/kg/d rasburicase until clinical response shows recovery Allopurinol is not the drug of choice for TLS unless patient has G6PD deficiency or allergy to rasburicase
1C. Strongly recommended based on low-quality evidence	Establish a multidisciplinary team (hematology, nephrology, intensivists) to manage patient care If appropriate intensive care staff and facilities are not available, consider transferring patient to achieve this level of care Do not alkalinize the urine Symptomatic hypocalcemia should be treated with calcium gluconate in standard doses for age/weight, carefully monitoring calcium, phosphate, and renal function Peritoneal dialysis is not recommended for TLS
2C. Weak recommendation based on low-quality evidence	Asymptomatic hypocalcemia should not be treated Hyperkalemia $\geq$6.0 mmol/L or >25% increase above baseline should have cardiac monitoring

Adapted from Jones GL, Will A, Jackson GH, et al. Guidelines for the management of tumour lysis syndrome in adults and children with haematological malignancies on behalf of the British Committee for Standards in Haematology. Br J Haematol 2015;169(5):661–71; with permission.

MANAGEMENT OF ACUTE HYPERURICEMIA

Treatment of hyperuricemia begins with aggressive hydration to maintain high urine output.[12] Balanced or isotonic solutions administered at 3 L/m² every 24 hours inhibit uric acid and calcium phosphate deposits in the renal tubules.[13,29] These solutions should not be supplemented with potassium because it can worsen hyperkalemia and lead to cardiac arrhythmias.[13] Urine alkalinization is also avoided because it increases calcium phosphate precipitation, and decreases the solubility of xanthine, an intermediate metabolite of uric acid.[12] Monitoring fluid intake and losses no less frequently than every 6 hours quantifies fluid balance and can predict potential fluid overload, especially for patients with preexisting renal or cardiac disease.

Pharmacologic treatment of hyperuricemia includes rasburicase and, in special situations, allopurinol.[12] Each agent is indicated for separate scenarios because of their different mechanisms of action. Rasburicase is a urate oxidase, an enzyme that actively metabolizes uric acid to allantoin, which is water soluble.[12] When administered as a 30-minute infusion, rasburicase reduces uric acid levels faster than allopurinol. Rasburicase should be offered to all high-risk adults and children in single doses as prophylaxis before treatment, and to patients with symptomatic TLS at 0.2 mg/kg/d unless contraindicated.[12] The duration of treatment is between 3 to 7 days depending on the patient's response. Rasburicase is rated as pregnancy class C (animal studies have shown adverse effects on the fetus and no well-controlled human studies are available) and severe allergic reactions, including anaphylaxis, have been reported.

Rasburicase is contraindicated in patients with glucose-6-phosphate dehydrogenase (G6PD) deficiency whose erythrocytes respond poorly to oxidative stress. The strong oxidizing agent hydrogen peroxide is a by-product of uric acid metabolism and can trigger severe hemolysis if rasburicase is administered to G6PD-deficient patients. As a genetic disorder, G6PD deficiency may affect up to 10% of African American men in the United States, thus, formal testing for G6PD deficiency is recommended before initiating rasburicase in patients with African or Mediterranean descent.[30,31] Rasburicase may also cause methemoglobinemia and serious hypoxemia, which is typically treated with intravenous methylene blue. However, multiple case studies have reported the development of refractory methemoglobinemia as a result of this adverse effect of rasburicase combined with an undiagnosed G6PD deficiency.[32–36] Because intravenous methylene blue is the treatment of choice for methemoglobinemia, and it is contraindicated in G6PD deficiency; treatment of TLS in G6PD-deficient patients must exclude rasburicase, and is limited to allopurinol and symptom management.[30]

Allopurinol attenuates uric acid production by inhibiting xanthine oxidase; however, it has no effect on existing uric acid deposits in the renal tubules.[2] Allopurinol should only be administered prophylactically to intermediate-risk patients 48 hours before antineoplastic treatment at a dose of 100 mg/m^2 every 8 hours.[1,28] Higher doses or a switch to rasburicase may be necessary if biochemical markers do not improve.[12] Otherwise, as noted earlier, it is reserved for the treatment of TLS in G6PD-deficient patients.

Treatment of Hyperphosphatemia and Hypocalcemia

The abundant discharge of nucleic acids, proteins, and metabolites from tumor cells into the bloodstream produces hyperphosphatemia ($\geq$6.5 mg/dL [2.1 mmol/L] in children, >4.48 mg/dL [1.45 mmol/L] in adults, or 25% increase from baseline). Fluid hydration and uricosuric drugs can treat hyperphosphatemia by improving renal excretion of phosphate. A phosphate-restricted diet and aluminum hydroxide at 50 to 150 mg/kg/d has been recommended.[1] However, aluminum hydroxide has a slow onset and dialysis is indicated if all other measures fail.[1,11]

Treatment of hypocalcemia ($\leq$7 mg/dL [1.75 mmol/L] or 25% decrease from baseline) is only indicated when it is symptomatic, because of the risk of accelerating calcium phosphate deposits in the renal tubules. A 1000-mg calcium gluconate infusion can treat hypocalcemia-related first-degree atrioventricular block, widened QRS, seizures, and tetany.[1,11] Patients with TLS with asymptomatic hypocalcemia should have continuous cardiac monitoring for electrocardiographic changes but should not be treated with exogenous calcium.

Treatment of Hyperkalemia

Hyperkalemia (>6 mEq/L [6.0 mmol/L] or 25% increase from baseline) necessitates cardiac monitoring because it can lead to cardiac arrhythmias and death. Loop diuretics can treat hyperkalemia by inhibiting potassium reabsorption at the loop of Henle.[1] However, loop diuretics should be administered judiciously because furosemide can precipitate uric acid crystallization in the renal tubules.[2] Injection of 10 units of regular insulin can shift potassium ions intracellularly; 50% dextrose should be administered concurrent with insulin treatment to prevent hypoglycemia.[1] Nebulized albuterol, a selective β2-adrenergic agonist, promotes the intracellular shift of potassium ions.[1] However, nearly 40% of patients with compromised renal function are resistant to the potassium level–lowering effect of albuterol, and it is not possible to predict the responders from the nonresponders.[37] Administering insulin and albuterol together can synergistically decrease plasma potassium concentration by about 1.2 mmol/L after 1 hour.[37] A calcium gluconate infusion can stabilize cardiac myocytes and prevent developing cardiac arrhythmias, although it has no direct effect on serum potassium level.[1]

Dialysis is recommended if electrolyte derangements are refractory to treatment or life threatening, which becomes more likely in the setting of volume overload or renal insufficiency. Because of the highly proliferative nature of tumor cells, and the continual release of solute into the blood stream, daily dialysis is recommended until the crisis passes.[29] However, patients who are hemodynamically unstable and refractory to pharmacologic treatment benefit from continuous renal replacement therapy.[29]

SUMMARY

TLS is a life-threatening disorder that is classified as an oncologic emergency. Risk factors for TLS are well known, but the current literature is replete with case descriptions of unexpected acute TLS. It is now known that solid tumors and untreated hematologic tumors can lyse under various circumstances in both children and adults. International guidelines and recommendations, including the early involvement of the critical care team, have been put forward to help clinicians properly manage the syndrome. Advanced practice nurses may be in the position of both triaging and initiating treatment of patients with TLS, and therefore need a thorough understanding of the syndrome and its treatment.

REFERENCES

1. Lewis MA, Hendrickson AW, Moynihan TJ. Oncologic emergencies: pathophysiology, presentation, diagnosis, and treatment. CA Cancer J Clin 2011;61(5): 287–314.
2. Will A, Tholouli E. The clinical management of tumour lysis syndrome in haematological malignancies. Br J Haematol 2011;154:3–13.
3. McBride A, Westervelt P. Recognizing and managing the expanded risk of tumor lysis syndrome in hematologic and solid malignancies. J Hematol Oncol 2012;5:75.
4. Ayed S, Bornstain C, Vincent F. Evolving concepts in tumour lysis syndrome management. Br J Haematol 2016;173(3):485–6.
5. Lipkowitz MS. Regulation of uric acid excretion by the kidney. Curr Rheumatol Rep 2012;14(2):179–88.
6. Bobulescu IA, Moe OW. Renal transport of uric acid: evolving concepts and uncertainties. Adv Chronic Kidney Dis 2012;19(6):358–71.
7. Wilson FP, Berns JS. Tumor lysis syndrome: New challenges and recent advances. Adv Chronic Kidney Dis 2014;21(1):18–26.
8. Ejaz AA, Pourafshar N, Mohandas R, et al. Uric acid and the prediction models of tumor lysis syndrome in AML. PLoS One 2015;10(3):e0119497.
9. Flombaum CD. Metabolic emergencies in the cancer patient. Semin Oncol 2000; 27:322–34.
10. Zusman J, Brown DM, Nesbit ME. Hyperphosphatemia, hyperphosphaturia and hypocalcemia in acute lymphoblastic leukemia. N Engl J Med 1973;289:1335–40.
11. Chang WT, Radin B, McCurdy MT. Calcium, magnesium, and phosphate abnormalities in the emergency department. Emerg Med Clin North Am 2014;32(2): 349–66.

12. Jones GL, Will A, Jackson GH, et al. Guidelines for the management of tumour lysis syndrome in adults and children with haematological malignancies on behalf of the British Committee for Standards in Haematology. Br J Haematol 2015; 169(5):661–71.

13. Cairo MS, Bishop M. Tumour lysis syndrome: new therapeutic strategies and classification. Br J Haematol 2004;127(1):3–11.

14. Van Der Klooster JM, Van Der Wiel HE, Van Saase JL, et al. Asystole during combination chemotherapy for non-Hodgkin's lymphoma: the acute tumor lysis syndrome. Neth J Med 2000;56(4):147–52.

15. Alfarouk KO, Verduzco D, Rauch C, et al. Glycolysis, tumor metabolism, cancer growth and dissemination. A new pH-based etiopathogenic perspective and therapeutic approach to an old cancer question. Oncoscience 2014;1(12): 777–802.

16. Gallo M, Sapio L, Spina A, et al. Lactic dehydrogenase and cancer: an overview. Front Biosci (Landmark Ed) 2015;20:1234–49.

17. Brown JE, Cook RJ, Lipton A, et al. Serum lactate dehydrogenase is prognostic for survival in patients with bone metastases from breast cancer: a retrospective analysis in bisphosphonate-treated patients. Clin Cancer Res 2012;18(22): 6348–55.

18. Miao P, Sheng S, Sun X, et al. Lactate dehydrogenase A in cancer: a promising target for diagnosis and therapy. IUBMB Life 2013;65(11):904–10.

19. Augoff K, Hryniewicz-Jankowska A, Tabola R. Lactate dehydrogenase 5: an old friend and a new hope in the war on cancer. Cancer Lett 2015;358(1):1–7.

20. Kim HS, Lee HE, Yang HK, et al. High lactate dehydrogenase 5 expression correlates with high tumoral and stromal vascular endothelial growth factor expression in gastric cancer. Pathobiology 2014;81(2):78–85.

21. Daly GF, Barnard EB, Thoreson L. Renal calculi: an unusual presentation of T-cell acute lymphoblastic leukemia. Pediatrics 2016;137(1):e20143877.

22. Shenoy MT, D'Souza B, Akshatha LN, et al. spontaneous tumor lysis syndrome in an infant: a case report. Indian J Clin Biochem 2015;30(3):360–2.

23. Chubb EA, Maloney D, Farley-Hills E. Tumour lysis syndrome: an unusual presentation. Anaesthesia 2010;65:1031–3.

24. Sinha R, Bose S, Subramaniam R. Tumor lysis under anesthesia in a child. Acta Anaesthesiol Scand 2009;53(1):131–3.

25. McDonnell C, Barlow R, Campisi P, et al. Fatal peri-operative acute tumour lysis syndrome precipitated by dexamethasone. Anaesthesia 2008;63(6):652–5.

26. Lee MH, Cheng KI, Jang RC, et al. Tumour lysis syndrome developing during an operation. Anaesthesia 2007;62:85–7.

27. Duzova A, Cetin M, Gumruk F, et al. Acute tumour lysis syndrome following a single-dose corticosteroid in children with acute lymphoblastic leukaemia. Eur J Haematol 2001;66:404–7.

28. Guyatt G, Oxman AD, Akl EA, et al. GRADE guidelines: 1. Introduction-GRADE evidence profiles and summary of findings tables. J Clin Epidemiol 2011;64(4): 383–94.

29. Tosi P, Barosi G, Lazzaro C, et al. Consensus conference on the management of tumor lysis syndrome. Haematologica 2008;93:1877–85.

30. Relling MV, McDonagh EM, Chang T, et al. Clinical Pharmacogenetics Implementation Consortium. Clinical Pharmacogenetics Implementation Consortium (CPIC) guidelines for rasburicase therapy in the context of G6PD deficiency genotype. Clin Pharmacol Ther 2014;96(2):169–74.

31. Glucose-6-dehydrogenase deficiency. Available at: https://ghr.nlm.nih.gov/condition/glucose-6-phosphate-dehydrogenase-deficiency#. Accessed June 28, 2016.

32. Alessa MA, Craig AK, Cunningham JM. Rasburicase-induced methemoglobinemia in a patient with aggressive non-Hodgkin's lymphoma. Am J Case Rep 2015;16:590–3.

33. Montgomery KW, Booth GS. A perfect storm: Tumor lysis syndrome with rasburicase-induced methemoglobinemia in a G6PD deficient adult. J Clin Apher 2017;32(1):62–3.

34. Roberts DA, Freed JA. Rasburicase-induced methemoglobinemia in two African-American female patients: an under-recognized and continued problem. Eur J Haematol 2015;94(1):83–5.

35. Bontant T, Le Garrec S, Avran D, et al. Methaemoglobinaemia in a G6PD-deficient child treated with rasburicase. BMJ Case Rep 2014. http://dx.doi.org/10.1136/bcr-2014-204706.

36. Cheah CY, Lew TE, Seymour JF, et al. Rasburicase causing severe oxidative hemolysis and methemoglobinemia in a patient with previously unrecognized glucose-6-phosphate dehydrogenase deficiency. Acta Haematol 2013;130(4):254–9.

37. Weisberg LS. Management of severe hyperkalemia. Crit Care Med 2008;36(12):3246–51.

Neurologic Intensive Care Unit Electrolyte Management

Craig Hutto, BSN, MSN, AGACNP-BC*, Mindy French, BSN, MSN, ACNP-BC*

KEYWORDS

- Dysnatremia • Hyponatremia • Hypernatremia • Neurologic surgery • Intensive care

KEY POINTS

- Alterations in sodium levels are common among intensive care patients, and have been associated with poor outcomes in certain intracranial processes.
- Differentiating between the syndrome of inappropriate antidiuretic hormone and cerebral salt wasting is imperative in the correct treatment of neurologic intensive care patients.
- Diabetes insipidus is a common postsurgical finding following pituitary surgery.

DEFINITION

Dysnatremia is a common finding in the intensive care unit (ICU) and has been suggested to be a predictor for mortality and poor clinical outcomes.[1–3] Depending on the time of onset (ie, on admission vs later in the ICU stay), the incidence of dysnatremias in critically ill patients ranges from 6.9% to 15%, respectively.[4,5] The symptoms of sodium derangement and their effect on brain physiology make early recognition and correction paramount in the neurologic ICU (NICU). Hyponatremia in brain injured patients can lead to life-threatening conditions such as seizures and may worsen cerebral edema and contribute to alterations in intracranial pressure.[6]

DIAGNOSIS

Critical illness may result in activity fluctuations of antidiuretic hormone.[7,8] Patients with certain neurologic diseases, such as subarachnoid hemorrhages or traumatic brain injuries, are at an additional risk of dysnatremias. The patient population in an NICU are widespread and include, but are not limited to, traumatic brain injuries (TBIs), hemorrhagic and ischemic strokes, neoplasms, and infections; each has its own prevalence for sodium alterations (**Box 1**). For example, neurosurgery (specifically transsphenoidal pituitary surgery) has an incidence of postoperative diabetes insipidus (DI) that ranges from 1.6% to 31%.[9–11] The incidence of hypernatremia

Department of Anesthesiology and Perioperative Medicine, Oregon Health and Science University, 3181 SW Sam Jackson Road, Portland, OR 97239, USA
* Corresponding author.
E-mail addresses: hutto@ohsu.edu; frencmi@ohsu.edu

Nurs Clin N Am 52 (2017) 321–329
http://dx.doi.org/10.1016/j.cnur.2017.01.009
0029-6465/17/© 2017 Elsevier Inc. All rights reserved.

nursing.theclinics.com

Box 1
Common causes of hypernatremia and hyponatremia in neurologically critically ill patients

Traumatic brain injury

Infections
  Meningitis
  Encephalitis

Neurovascular
  Thrombotic or embolic stroke
  Hemorrhagic stroke

Neoplasm
  Pituitary adenoma
  Meningioma
  Germinoma

Adapted from Faridi AB, Weisberg LS. Acid-base, electrolyte, and metabolic abnormalities. In: Parrillo JE, Dellinger, RP, editors. Critical care medicine: principles of diagnosis and management in the adult. 3rd edition. Philadelphia: Mosby; 2008. p. 1225.

---

following TBI ranges from 16% to 40%, whereas the prevalence of dysnatremias in aneurysmal subarachnoid hemorrhage (SAH) can range from 19% to 30%.[12,13] Distinguishing disorders affecting specifically the hypothalamic-neurohypophyseal system (ie, pituitary neoplasm/surgery) is important in diagnosis, duration, and management compared with systemic brain processes such as hemorrhagic strokes or TBI.

HYPERNATREMIA

Hypernatremia in critical illness has numerous causes and can be multifactorial. The diagnostic approach when dealing with dysnatremias should focus on the patient's volume status.[2,4,13] This article discusses euvolemic hypernatremia; specifically, DI.

Tonicity refers to the effect of plasma on cells. Hypernatremia always indicates hypertonicity, which results in cell shrinkage.[14] Plasma hypertonicity is a powerful stimulus for thirst (polydipsia), but, in acute brain injury, oral intake may be limited because of a decline in mental status.

DI is characterized by polydipsia and polyuria leading to an imbalance of water in the body. It can be caused by the decreased secretion of antidiuretic hormone (ADH), also known as central DI (CDI) or by a lack of renal responsiveness to the hormone, termed nephrogenic DI.[15] Providers in the NICU commonly come into contact with the neurologic form, CDI, which affects the hypothalamic-neurohypophyseal system. Clinical manifestations of CDI include large amounts of dilute urine, causing hypernatremia if the patient is unable to match the total fluid losses with water intake. The degree of the symptoms is proportional to the magnitude of the increase in sodium concentrations in the plasma, with chronic hypernatremia having milder symptoms than acute hypernatremia. Patients with chronic hypernatremia may experience weakness and lethargy, whereas acute hypernatremia may present as acute-onset headache, seizures, and even coma.[14,16]

CDI may follow 1 of 3 pathways following neurosurgery: either transient, permanent, or following a triphasic pattern. The first 2 phases occur in 2.7% to 13.6% of patients whereas the triphasic pattern has been described to occur in 3.4% of patients undergoing transsphenoidal pituitary surgery.[11,17] The pathophysiology of the triphasic phase begins with early hypothalamic dysfunction and inhibition of ADH resulting in polyuria, typically lasting 4 to 5 days. Second, there is release of the stored hormone, vasopressin, resulting in increasing urine osmolality. The third phase can become permanent CDI if all vasopressin stores are depleted.[18]

DIAGNOSIS OF DIABETES INSIPIDUS

DI is a clinical diagnosis that can be confirmed with laboratory tests. Clinical features include thirst and polyuria, which can be defined as urinary excretion of greater than 2.5 L in 24 hours for 2 consecutive days.[19] Postsurgical DI typically presents in the first 24 to 48 hours following surgery.[10] A common approach in the ICU setting for initiating serum and urine electrolyte testing is the presence of greater than 300 mL/h of urine for 2 consecutive hours and a specific gravity of less than 1.005. Laboratory findings are consistent with hypernatremia (>145 mmol/L), serum hyperosmolality, and hypoosmolar urine (Table 1).[15,16] Frequent biochemical analysis following surgery is suggested if postoperative DI is suspected.

TREATMENT OF DIABETES INSIPIDUS

The goal for treating CDI is focusing on restoring the body's normal osmotic homeostasis.[19] The patient should be allowed to drink to thirst, but, if unable to keep up with fluid losses, additional measures should be taken. The isotonic solution (hypotonic once in the body), 5% dextrose in water, can be given intravenously to match the total output.[20] If permanent DI is suspected or serum and urine electrolytes continue to be disrupted despite oral and/or intravenous fluids, ADH should be administered. The synthetic analogue of ADH is called desmopressin (desamino-D-arginine vasopressin [DDAVP]) and can administered intravenously, subcutaneously, nasally, and less frequently orally.[21] Hormone replacement in permanent DI reduces urine output, thereby improving homeostasis.

HYPONATREMIA

Hyponatremia has been shown to occur in up to 30% of ICU patients and is one of the most common electrolyte disorders.[22] Hyponatremia is the most common electrolyte abnormality in patients with aneurysmal subarachnoid hemorrhage, occurring in 35%

Table 1
Comparison of diabetes insipidus, syndrome of inappropriate antidiuretic hormone secretion, and cerebral salt wasting pituitary disorders

	DI	SIADH	CSW
Urine Output	↑↑	Normal	↑↑
Serum Sodium	↑↑	↓↓	↓↓
Urine Sodium	↓	↑↑	↑↑
Serum Osmolality	↑↑	↓↓	↓↓
Urine Osmolality	↓↓	↑↑	↑↑
Serum Uric Acid (Before Sodium Correction)	↑↑	↓/Normal	↓↓
Excretion of Uric Acid (Before Sodium Correction)	↓↓	↑↑	↑↑
Serum Uric Acid (After Sodium Correction)	↑↑	Normal	↓↓
Excretion of Uric Acid (After Sodium Correction)	↓↓	Normal	↓↓
Urine Specific Gravity	↓↓	↑↑	Normal
Fluid Volume Status	↓↓	Normal	↓↓

to 50% of cases.[23,24] The clinical manifestations of hyponatremia can range from anorexia, headache, nausea, vomiting, lethargy, and seizures in severe cases.[15] Symptoms are attributed to cellular edema, which occurs in hypotonic hyponatremia, and can have grave consequences such as increased intracranial pressure. It has been associated with an increase in mortality in patients with intracranial hemorrhages.[25,26] There are numerous causal factors associated with hyponatremia in the acute care setting, depending on tonicity and volume status.[27] Classification of hyponatremia can be based on plasma osmolality, volume status, and urine tonicity (**Box 2**). This article first focuses on euvolemic hyponatremia caused by the syndrome of inappropriate antidiuretic hormone (SIADH) as it relates to the neurologic population, and then it discusses hypovolemic hyponatremia caused by cerebral salt wasting (CSW) syndrome in patients with aneurysmal subarachnoid hemorrhage.

Most hyponatremias are associated with hypo-osmolality. In general, this is caused by an increase in water intake and/or a decrease of renal water excretion. Water excretion impaired by failure to suppress the superfluous release of ADH is termed SIADH.[15] Patients with SIADH have low sodium levels, hypo-osmolality, and concentrated urine. There is a similar form of hyponatremia in patients with brain diseases, called CSW, in which there is loss of sodium in the urine. The cause of CSW is not fully understood, and remains a controversial topic following brain injury.[28] The distinction between the two disorders relies on volume status. In CSW, increased ADH secretion results in volume depletion, compared with patients with SIADH who remain euvolemic.[15,16] The distinction between the two syndromes becomes important in the clinical setting because they require different treatments.[29] This distinction becomes important in the treatment of subarachnoid hemorrhages, which should not be fluid restricted, because of the risk of vasospasm.[30,31]

ASSESSMENT AND TREATMENT
Syndrome of Inappropriate Antidiuretic Hormone

In the setting of normal kidney and liver function (and exclusion of hypothyroidism/central adrenal insufficiency), SIADH has biochemical findings consisting of hyponatremia, plasma hypo-osmolality, and urine sodium level greater than 30 mmol/L.[32] Frequent assessment of serum and urine electrolytes, total intake, and urinary output should be performed when treating SIADH.[15,16] Although correction of the underlying cause is needed, the mainstay treatment of SIADH relies on water intake restriction.[15] Water restriction has been shown to improve patients to normonatremia after subarachnoid hemorrhage; however, hypovolemia should be avoided in this population.[33] Patients unable to achieve correction with water restriction or isotonic saline may be candidates for demeclocycline or conivaptan.[16] Ultimately, sodium correction depends on the acuity of sodium alterations; thus, patients with asymptomatic hyponatremia do not need aggressive correction.[15]

Box 2
Classification of hyponatremia

- Isotonic hyponatremia
- Hypertonic hyponatremia
- Hypotonic hyponatremia
  - Euvolemic hyponatremia
  - Hypervolemic hyponatremia
  - Hypovolemic hyponatremia

Cerebral Salt Wasting

CSW is a complicated pathophysiologic condition defined as a hypovolemic hyponatremia that is most commonly seen in patients with aneurysmal subarachnoid hemorrhage (aSAH).[31] The cause of CSW remains unknown; however, there are several mechanisms that are suspected to play a role in CSW. Differentiating CSW from SIADH is imperative when developing a treatment regimen, because the two syndromes are treated differently.[24,31] The difference between CSW and SIADH is based on the patient's volume status.[34] In CSW, patients are hypovolemic, whereas in SIADH the patients are euvolemic to hypervolemic.[23,24]

The pathophysiology of CSW is poorly understood. The diagnosis of CSW was originally identified in the 1950s by Peters and colleagues.[35] Later studies in the late 1950s identified the syndrome of inappropriate ADH secretion.[36] There have been a vast number of studies performed in an attempt to understand the underlying cause of CSW. Several theories currently exist to explain CSW in brain-injured patients, including sympathetic nervous system dysfunction, alteration in the renin-angiotensin-aldosterone system (RAAS) pathway, and natriuretic peptide influence.[23,31,37]

The mechanism of action for natriuresis and diuresis in CSW is largely unknown. Some studies suggest that natriuretic peptides could play a role in the water and sodium dysregulation that can be seen in patients with aSAH. Atrial natriuretic peptide (ANP) and brain natriuretic peptide (BNP) have been associated with disruptions in water and sodium balance in aSAH and additional research is ongoing. The RAAS is a hormonal pathway that regulates total body sodium and water. Renin is an enzyme that is released when there is low renal arterial perfusion. Its release initiates multiple enzymes, including angiotensin-converting enzyme, which produces angiotensin II (AT II). AT II is a potent vasoconstrictor, which immediately goes to work on the peripheral vasculature, increasing blood pressure and stimulating the release of ADH. AT II stimulates the release of aldosterone, which is instrumental in the maintenance of fluid volume and sodium and potassium concentrations in the body. There have been studies that suggest that there may be a cerebrally mediated activation of the RAAS, and that there could be cerebral intrinsic AT II, which could result in increased sympathetic tone in the peripheral vascular system.[31]

It is widely known that the sympathetic nervous system plays a vital role in sodium and water regulation, as described earlier. A controversial theory related to the disruption of the central nervous system (CNS) and its potential alteration in renal salt and water regulation also exists. The idea behind this theory is that specific renal innervation is altered during CNS injury. This alteration could potentially decrease adrenergic tone to the kidney, which in turn could lead to a decrease in renin secretion and a subsequent decreased level of circulating aldosterone. These enzymatic and hormonal changes could contribute to decreased sodium and water reabsorption, creating fluid and sodium excretion. This theory is flawed in that there is overwhelming evidence that severe CNS injury causes a sympathetic surge, as shown by the presence of stress cardiomyopathy and neurogenic pulmonary edema. It is difficult to conceptualize the idea that specific organ systems (heart and lungs) could see an increase in sympathetic activity, whereas others (kidneys) could experience a decrease in adrenergic tone. Studies are ongoing in an attempt to more intricately understand the autonomic nervous system's response to CNS injury.[31]

In the 1980s, natriuretic peptides were discovered. Natriuretic peptides are molecules that normally defend against periods of excess water and salt retention by antagonizing the RAAS.[31] Since that time, several specific natriuretic substances have been identified and studied. With regard to CSW, there have been 4 main natriuretic peptides that have been identified.[38] ANP, BNP, C-type natriuretic peptide (CNP), and dendroaspis natriuretic peptide (DNP). All 4 of the peptides have specific tissue site production. ANP and DNP are predominantly found in atrial myocardial muscles, BNP in the ventricles of the heart, and CNP in the telencephalon, hypothalamus, and endothelium. All of the peptides cause relaxation of vascular smooth muscle resulting in dilatation of veins and arteries. The effect on the nephron is an increase in filtration of water and sodium through the glomerulus, which can lead to hypovolemia and hyponatremia. These peptides have direct effect on the renal tubule by inhibiting angiotensin-induced resorption of sodium and by antagonizing the action of vasopressin at the collecting ducts. In the adrenal medulla, there is production and release of natriuretic peptides that can potentially have paracrine inhibitory effects on mineralocorticoid synthesis. This process could explain why there is not an increase in aldosterone and renin levels in patients with CSW who are hypovolemic.[31]

In a study by McGirt and colleagues[37], levels of BNP were found in patients with SAH and there was a relationship between high BNP levels and low serum sodium levels. Unusually high levels of BNP also correlated with cerebral vasospasm. It is possible that the initial CNS insult of aneurysmal rupture into the subarachnoid space could cause release of BNP from damage to the cortical and subcortical structures in which BNP exists.[31] Some studies suggest that BNP released from the hypothalamus in the setting of CNS injury could be a protective mechanism to decrease intracranial pressure by inducing natriuresis. BNP seemed to be the primary natriuretic peptide that caused salt wasting in patients with SAH.[23] The surge of sympathetic flow at the onset of CNS injury is also likely responsible for the increased peptide levels caused by myocardial strain secondary to catecholamine release.

Additional research is warranted to help identify the mechanism of action of each of these peptides and their contribution to hypovolemia and hyponatremia consistent with CSW syndrome in patients with aneurysmal subarachnoid hemorrhage.

Diagnosis and Treatment of Cerebral Salt Wasting

Diagnosis of CSW relies heavily on accurate fluid volume assessment. Several studies have been conducted in an attempt to identify the most accurate method with which to assess fluid volume balance in the ICU.[39] Central venous pressure is a common method of assessment, but has been proved to be unreliable.[40] Many studies have compared volume indices between pulmonary artery catheterization (PAC) and transpulmonary thermodilution measurements (pulse-index contour cardiac output [PiCCO]). One study showed successful volume management and a decrease in complications with the use of PiCCO compared with the use of PAC.[41]

When assessing laboratory data, patients with SIADH have serum uric acid levels and fractional excretion of uric acid that become normal once the sodium level is corrected. In patients with CSW, uric acid levels stay low and uric acid excretion remains increased even after sodium levels have been corrected.[23] Urine sodium, urine and serum osmolality, and volume status are key markers to evaluate when attempting to differential SIADH from CSW before correction of sodium level. However, it is not possible to differentiate between CSW and SIADH by evaluating urine and serum Na and osmolality alone.[31] Assessment of fluid volume status using PAC or PiCCO is recommended.

Once CSW is diagnosed, treatment of CSW should focus on fluid volume repletion to euvolemia and repletion of sodium deficit. Repletion of fluid deficit using normal saline is imperative, because hypovolemia has been associated with increased risk of vasospasm in patients with subarachnoid hemorrhage.[30,31] Blood volume analysis and PiCCO monitoring should be used to guide volume repletion in an attempt to prevent hypervolemia, which has been associated with poor outcomes in patients with subarachnoid hemorrhage.[38] Once euvolemia has been restored, the focus should turn to sodium repletion. There is evidence that there is an alteration in the hypothalamic-pituitary axis in patients with aSAH and, in turn, a mineralocorticoid deficiency. Using mineralocorticoid replacement with fludrocortisone can also be effective in patients with aSAH and CSW. Fludrocortisone treatment reduces the incidence of hyponatremia without developing serious consequences of fluid overload. Hypertonic saline can also be useful in correction of hyponatremia, especially when sodium levels are dangerously low (<125 mEq/L).[31] Sodium levels should be assessed frequently during hypertonic therapy to prevent rapid overcorrection, such as myelinolysis.[31] Sodium correction should not exceed 0.5 mEq/h and the target sodium goal should be normonatremia (135–145 mEq/L).[31] Potassium levels should also be checked frequently because of the risk of hypokalemia with the use of fludrocortisone.[42]

SUMMARY

Alterations in serum sodium levels are common among critically ill patients, and may worsen outcomes if not recognized and managed appropriately. Certain dysnatremias have higher incidences in acutely brain injured patients, and have been associated with higher mortality. Before any treatment ensues, clinicians must diagnose the problem. A serum sodium level that is greater than or less than the reference range should warrant further investigation, including assessment of plasma and urine tonicity, frequent monitoring of urinary output, and evaluation of the patient's volume status. For patients with hypernatremia caused by DI, the mainstay treatment is replacement of fluid losses, either by having the patient drink to thirst or by administering intravenous isotonic solutions in some situations. In permanent DI, hormone replacement is needed to reduce urinary output, thereby improving homeostasis.

Hyponatremia in neurologically ill patients may have serious consequences if not treated correctly. This article discusses SIADH and CSW, which ultimately are distinguished by the patient's volume status. It is important to have the correct diagnosis, because the treatments are opposite. Management of SIADH relies on fluid restrictions, whereas the patient with CSW needs fluid repletion. However, practitioners must be cognizant of fluid restrictions in patients with subarachnoid hemorrhage with SIADH, because hypovolemia can worsen vasospasms.

The dynamic environment of the ICU can make diagnosis and treatment of critically ill patients challenging. The NICU is a perfect example of a dynamic environment. There are numerous studies on dysnatremias in neurologic critical care that have the potential to improve outcomes, making it vital to be familiar with the current literature.

REFERENCES

1. Beseoglu K, Etminan N, Steiger HJ, et al. The relationship of early hypernatremia with clinical outcome in patients suffering from aneurysmal subarachnoid hemorrhage. Clin Neurol Neurosurg 2014;123:164–8.

2. Bennani SL, Abouqal R, Zeggwagh AA, et al. Incidence, causes and prognostic factors of hyponatremia in an intensive care unit. Rev Med Interne 2003;24:224–9.

3. Polderman KH, Schreuder WO, van Schijndel RJ, et al. Hypernatremia in the intensive care unit: an indicator of quality of care? Crit Care Med 1999;27(6):1105–8.

4. Oude Lansink-Hartgring A, Hessels L, Weigel J, et al. Long-term changes in dysnatremia incidence in the ICU: a shift from hyponatremia to hypernatremia. Ann Intensive Care 2016;6(22):1–8.

5. Funk GC, Lindner G, Druml W, et al. Incidence and prognosis of dysnatremias present on ICU admission. Intensive Care Med 2010;36:304–11.

6. Brimioulle S, Orellana-Jimenez C, Aminian A, et al. Hyponatremia in neurological patients: cerebral salt wasting versus inappropriate antidiuretic hormone secretion. Intensive Care Med 2008;34:125–31.

7. Jochberger S, Mayr VD, Luckner G, et al. Serum vasopressin concentrations in critically ill patients. Crit Care Med 2006;34:293–9.

8. Siami S, Bailly-Salin J, Polito A, et al. Osmoregulation of vasopressin secretion is altered in the postacute phase of septic shock. Crit Care Med 2010;38:1962–9.

9. Black PM, Zervas NT, Candia GL. Incidence and management of complications of transsphenoidal operation for pituitary adenomas. Neurosurgery 1987;20(6): 920–4.

10. Singer PA, Sevilla LJ. Postoperative endocrine management of pituitary tumors. Neurosurg Clin N Am 2003;14(1):123–38.

11. Hensen J, Henig A, Fahlbusch R, et al. Prevalence, predictors and patterns of postoperative polyuria and hyponatremia in the immediate course after transsphenoidal surgery for pituitary adenomas. Clin Endocrinol (Oxf) 1999;50:431–9.

12. Kolmodin L, Sekhon MS, Henderson WR, et al. Hypernatremia in patients with severe traumatic brain injury: a systematic review. Ann Intensive Care 2013;3(35): 1–7.

13. Qureshi AI, Suri FK, Sung GY, et al. Prognostic significance of hypernatremia and hyponatremia among patients with aneurysmal subarachnoid hemorrhage. Neurosurgery 2002;50(4):749–56.

14. Sterns RH. Disorders of plasma sodium – causes, consequences, and correction. N Engl J Med 2015;372:55–65.

15. Andreoli TE, Safirstein RL. Fluid and electrolyte disorders. In: Andreoli TE, Carpenter CC, Griggs RC, et al, editors. Cecil essentials of medicine. Philadelphia: Saunders; 2007. p. 289–92.

16. Faridi AB, Weisberg LS. Acid-base, electrolyte, and metabolic abnormalities. In: Parrillo JE, Dellinger RP, editors. Critical care medicine: principles of diagnosis and management in the adult. 3rd edition. Philadelphia: Mosby; 2008. p. 1219–26.

17. Sigounas DG, Sharpless JL, Cheng DM, et al. Predictors and incidence of central diabetes insipidus after endoscopic pituitary surgery. Neurosurgery 2008;62:71.

18. Hoorn EJ, Zietse R. Water balance disorders after neurosurgery: the triphasic response revisited. NDT Plus 2010;3:42–4.

19. Baylis PH, Thompson CJ. Diabetes insipidus and hyperosmolar syndromes. In: Becker KL, Bilezikian JP, Bremner WJ, editors. Principles and practice of endocrinology and metabolism. Philadelphia: Lippincott Williams & Wilkins; 2001. p. 285–93.

20. Capatina C, Paluzzi A, Mitchell R, et al. Diabetes insipidus after traumatic brain injury. J Clin Med 2015;4(7):1448–62.

21. Singer I, Oster JR, Fishman LM. The management of diabetes insipidus in adults. Arch Intern Med 1997;157(12):1293–301.

22. DeVita MV, Gardenswartz MH, Konecky A, et al. Incidence and etiology of hyponatremia in an intensive care unit. Clin Nephrol 1990;34(4):163–6.

23. Momi J, Tang C, Abcar A, et al. Hyponatremia–what is cerebral salt wasting? Perm J 2010;14(2):62–5.
24. Rabinstein AA, Bruder N. Management of hyponatremia and volume contraction. Neurocrit Care 2011;15(2):354–60.
25. Carcel C, Sato S, Zheng D, et al. Prognostic significance of hyponatremia in acute intracerebral hemorrhage: pooled analysis of the intensive blood pressure reduction in acute cerebral hemorrhage trial studies. Crit Care Med 2016;44(7): 1388–94.
26. Mapa B, Taylor BE, Appelboom G, et al. Impact of hyponatremia on morbidity, mortality, and complications after aneurysmal subarachnoid hemorrhage: a systematic review. World Neurosurg 2016;85:305–14.
27. Padhi R, Panda BN, Jagati S, et al. Hyponatremia in critically ill patients. Indian J Crit Care Med 2014;18(2):83–7.
28. Adler SM, Verbalis JG. Disorders of body water homeostasis in critical illness. Endocrinol Metab Clin North Am 2006;35:873–94.
29. Gritti P, Lanterna LA, Rotasperti L, et al. Clinical evaluation of hyponatremia and hypovolemia in critically ill adult neurologic patients: contribution of the use of cumulative balance of sodium. J Anesth 2014;28(5):687–95.
30. Diringer MN. Management of sodium abnormalities in patients with CNS disease. Clin Neuropharmacol 1992;15:427–47.
31. Yee AH, Burns JD, Wijdicks EF. Cerebral salt wasting: pathophysiology, diagnosis and treatment. Neurosurg Clin N Am 2010;21:339–52.
32. Cuesta M, Hannon MJ, Thompson CJ. Diagnosis and treatment of hyponatremia in neurosurgical patients. Endocrinol Nutr 2016;63(5):230–8.
33. Doczi T, Bende J, Huszka E, et al. Syndrome of inappropriate secretion of antidiuretic hormone after subarachnoid hemorrhage. Neurosurgery 1981;9(4):394–7.
34. Nathan BR. Cerebral correlates of hyponatremia. Neurocrit Care 2007;06:72–8.
35. Peters JP, Welt LG, Sins EA, et al. A salt-wasting syndrome associated with cerebral disease. Trans Assoc Am Physicians 1950;63:57–63.
36. Schwartz WB, Bennett W, Curelop S, et al. A syndrome of renal sodium loss and hyponatremia probably resulting from inappropriate secretion of antidiuretic hormone. Am J Med 1957;23(4):529–42.
37. McGirt MJ, Blessing R, Nimjee SM, et al. Correlation of serum brain natriuretic peptide with hyponatremia and delated ischemic neurological deficits after subarachnoid hemorrhage. Neurosurgery 2004;54(6):1369–73.
38. Martini RP, Deem S, Brown M, et al. The association between fluid balance and outcomes after subarachnoid hemorrhage. Neurocrit Care 2012;17:191.
39. Gress DR, Participants in the International Multi-disciplinary Consensus Conference on the Critical Care Management of Subarachnoid Hemorrhage. Monitoring of volume status after subarachnoid hemorrhage. Neurocrit Care 2011;15(2): 270–4.
40. Vespa P, The Participants in the International Multi-disciplinary Consensus Conference on the Critical Care Management of Subarachnoid Hemorrhage. SAH pituitary adrenal dysfunction. Neurocrit Care 2011;15:365.
41. Mutoh T, Kazumata K, Ishikawa T, et al. Performance of bedside transpulmonary thermodilution monitoring for goal-directed hemodynamic management after subarachnoid hemorrhage. Stroke 2009;40:2368–74.
42. Lehmann L, Bendel S, Uelinger DE. Randomized, double-blind trial of the edict of fluid composition electrolyte acid-base, and fluid homeostasis in patients early after subarachnoid hemorrhage. Neurocrit Care 2013;18:5–12.

Abdominal Compartment Syndrome as a Complication of Fluid Resuscitation

Bradley R. Harrell, DNP, APRN, ACNP-BC[a,b,*], Sarah Miller, PhD, RN[c]

KEYWORDS

- Fluid resuscitation • Damage control resuscitation • Crystalloid • Colloid
- Third spacing • Capillary leak • Intra-abdominal hypertension
- Abdominal compartment syndrome

KEY POINTS

- Fluid resuscitation is an important aspect of nurse care in maintaining a patient's hemodynamic stability.
- Excessive fluid resuscitation, particularly with crystalloids, increases the likelihood that multisystem complications occur.
- Third spacing and capillary leak can occur secondary to excessive fluid resuscitation.
- Intra-abdominal hypertension (IAH) and abdominal compartment syndrome (ACS) are lethal complications of excessive fluid resuscitation.
- Damage control resuscitation (DCR) and establishing acceptable and measurable endpoints for fluid resuscitation are necessary to reduce overall mortality.

INTRODUCTION/BACKGROUND

ACS has gained increased attention and significance in the literature in recent years, prompting regular revision and updating of practice and nursing management guidelines. Augmented growth of focused research on ACS and related intra-abdominal pressure (IAP) prompted the WSACS - The Abdominal Compartment Society to develop consensus definitions in 2006, with clinical practice guidelines and

Disclosure Statement: Dr B.R. Harrell is a regular content reviewer and item writer for Elsevier. He is regularly reimbursed for this work.
 a Loewenberg College of Nursing, University of Memphis, Community Health Building, Office 3525, 4055 North Park Loop, Memphis, TN 38152, USA; b Nursing Management Guidelines Workgroup for Intra-Abdominal Hypertension and Abdominal Compartment Syndrome, WSACS - the Abdominal Compartment Society, PO Box 980454, Richmond, VA 23298-0454, USA; c Medical University of South Carolina, College of Nursing, 99 Jonathan Lucas Street, MSC 160, Charleston, SC 29425-1600, USA
* Corresponding author. Loewenberg College of Nursing, Community Health Building, Office 3525, 4055 North Park Loop, Memphis, TN 38152.
E-mail address: bharrell@memphis.edu

Nurs Clin N Am 52 (2017) 331–338
http://dx.doi.org/10.1016/j.cnur.2017.01.010
0029-6465/17/© 2017 Elsevier Inc. All rights reserved.

recommendations for critical research needs following in 2007 and 2009, respectively. Most recently in 2013, the WSACS updated the 2006 definitions and 2007 management recommendations to include pediatric populations and more directed care management, including appropriate fluid resuscitation interventions in critically ill patients. Although the WSACS guidelines integrated the multiple causes of IAH/ACS, this article provides a focused overview of the pathophysiology and clinical correlation between the development of ACS and fluid resuscitation. It is vitally important for nurse clinicians to understand and interpret clinical signs of IAH/ACS and perform advanced assessments, acute management, and judicious fluid resuscitation to optimize patient outcomes and reduce overall mortality associated with ACS.

IAP has been of interest to health care providers for more than 100 years.[1] Initial evidence emerged from animal studies examining the relationship of IAP on respiration, organ function, and urine output.[2,3] These early findings were associated with postoperative complications of abdominal surgery, namely pneumoperitoneum, causing increased pressures within the abdominal cavity.[4] ACS was largely overlooked until the 1980s when Kron and colleagues[5] used the termed ACS. Although clinical examination is inaccurate to detect IAP, the bedside nurse clinician may measure IAP via several different methods, with intravesical (urinary bladder) pressure considered the most efficient and cost effective.[6–13] Increased IAP typically measures between 5 mm Hg and 7 mm Hg in critically ill adults and from 0 mm Hg to 5 mm Hg in otherwise healthy adults.

ABDOMINAL PERFUSION PRESSURE

Abdominal perfusion pressure (APP), a measure of visceral organ perfusion, is a predictor of abdominal organ perfusion as well as a possible guide for resuscitation measures. The APP, which is a surrogate of the intra-abdominal perfusion driving pressure, is obtained by subtracting the IAP from the mean arterial pressure (MAP) using the formula, APP = MAP − IAP. Cheatham and colleagues[14] concluded that APP was statistically superior to both MAP and intravesicular pressure in predicting survival from IAH/ACS, reporting that an APP of 60 mm Hg in patients with ACS was 98% sensitive in predicting survival in a population largely composed of trauma patients. The study also concluded that APP is a more accurate predictor of resuscitation than arterial lactate, MAP, arterial pH, base deficit, or IAP. Although WSACS does not currently recommend using APP to guide resuscitation of critically ill patients with IAH, interpretation from these findings suggest an ideal APP is a value greater than 60 mm Hg. IAH occurs when the IAP ranges between 12 mm Hg and 25 mm Hg. ACS is defined as a sustained IAP greater than 20 mm Hg that is associated with new organ dysfunction or failure.[15]

INTRA-ABDOMINAL HYPERTENSION AND ABDOMINAL COMPARTMENT SYNDROME PATHOPHYSIOLOGY
Causes

Interpreting the pathophysiology of IAH and ACS requires an understanding that the abdominal cavity is a closed compartment, similar to that of the cranium or muscle fascia. The peritoneal compartment is rigidly contained by the costal arch, spine, and pelvis and more flexibly by the abdominal wall and the diaphragm.[15] Considering the containment of a closed compartment, it is understandable that the abdominal cavity is particularly vulnerable to external compression and internal displacement (both solid anatomic and fluid based) leading to pressure shifts. IAH can result from any internal or external cause for elevation of pressure within the abdominal compartment. IAP is affected by extrinsic variables, including blunt abdominal trauma, pressure occurring outside the abdominal wall with abdominal burn eschar, third-space edema, or military antishock trousers. Intrinsic variables include solid organ volume, hollow viscera volume, ascites, blood, fluid, gravid uterus, or tumors within the abdominal cavity.[16]

Abdominal Compartment Syndrome Risk and Mortality

Nurse clinicians should be aware of the multiple causes and risk factors for developing ACS. More relevant risks include abdominal surgery, major trauma, major burns, acute pancreatitis, peritoneal dialysis, intra-abdominal pathology, acidosis, and polytransfusion of blood products.[15] The mortality associated with ACS has been reported as high as 80%.[17] The complexity of a patient's presentation, comorbid conditions, consideration of additional risk factors, and surgical intervention all play a role in determining mortality rate. Harrell and Melander[17] reported a strong correlation between massive fluid resuscitation and mortality in trauma patients who develop ACS.

Systemic Effects

With rising IAP and development of ACS, progressive hypoperfusion and ischemia of tissues trigger a positive feedback loop of proinflammatory cytokines, generation and release of oxygen free radicals, and a decrease in cellular production of adenosine triphosphate. As the toxic effects on cell membranes are further potentiated, multiple body systems are adversely affected (**Fig. 1**). The cardiovascular system is significantly

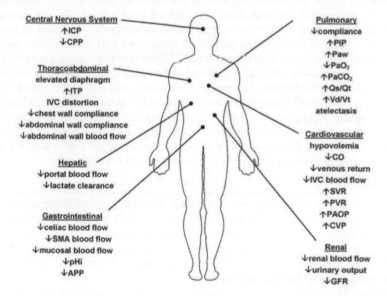

Fig. 1. Pathophysiologic effects of IAH and ACS. The effects of intra-abdominal hypertension are not limited just to the intra-abdominal organs, but rather have an impact either directly or indirectly on every organ system in the body. APP, abdominal perfusion pressure; CO, cardiac output; CPP, cerebral perfusion pressure; CVP, central venous pressure; GFR, glomerular filtration rate; ICP, intracranial pressure; ITP, intrathoracic pressure; IVC, inferior vena cava; $PaCO_2$, carbon dioxide tension; PaO_2, oxygen tension; PAOP, pulmonary artery occlusion pressure; Paw, mean airway pressure; pHi, gastric intramuscosal pH; PIP, peak inspiratory pressure; PVR, pulmonary vascular resistance; Qs/Qt, intrapulmonary shunt; SMA, superior mesenteric artery; SVR, systemic vascular resistance; Vd/Vt, pulmonary dead space. (*From* Cheatham ML. Abdominal compartment syndrome: pathophysiology and definitions. Scand J Trauma Resusc Emerg Med 2009;17:10.)

impacted by the increased abdominal pressure, which presses upward on the diaphragm, leading to secondary increased intrathoracic pressure. This increased intrathoracic pressure decreases venous return, resulting in reduced cardiac output and impairing homeostatic healing and perfusion capabilities.[16,18] Capillary leakage from inflammation continues to stimulate edema formation, and pulmonary wedge pressures and central venous pressures are increased, regardless of a patient's actual fluid volume status.[16] Additional cardiovascular effects include increased systemic vascular resistance and increased risk for venous thrombosis.[18] As pressures continue to rise in the thoracic cavity, resulting pulmonary effects include decreased lung compliance, increased peak inspiratory pressures, decreased Pao_2, increased $Paco_2$, and development of atelectasis.[16] Renal effects include decreased renal perfusion, decreased urinary output, and decreased glomerular filtration rates.[16] ACS affects multiple other organ systems including the hepatic, neurologic, and gastrointestinal systems. Because the multiple causes and massive systemic effects are beyond the scope of this article, the focus is on the risks associated with fluid resuscitation and subsequent cardiovascular, pulmonary, and renal compromise in patients that develop ACS.

FLUIDS AND DEVELOPMENT OF INTRA-ABDOMINAL HYPERTENSION/ABDOMINAL COMPARTMENT SYNDROME
Fluid Resuscitation

A notable risk factor for developing ACS is the use of aggressive fluid resuscitation, particularly in surgical, trauma, and burn patient populations. As previously discussed, the contained abdominal compartment is vulnerable to shifts in pressure and displacement of fluids. Initial guidelines suggested that resuscitation begin for all patients with crystalloid fluid resuscitation.[19] Prior to recent advancements in fluid resuscitation guidelines, critically ill patients were infused with several liters of crystalloid or colloid fluid in hopes of supporting circulatory and metabolic needs. Trauma providers primarily used crystalloids, whereas specific surgical cases may have used colloidal therapy. Aggressive infusion of crystalloids carries a risk of multiple complications, notably causing third-space edema in the abdominal cavity, increased IAP, IAH, and subsequent development of ACS. A more in-depth discussion follows to clarify the pathophysiology behind fluid movement and third spacing.

Fluid Movement

Inside the lumen of the capillary, the endothelial glycocalyx layer functions to produce an oncotic pressure to control the movement of fluids through the capillaries.[20] Initially, the movement of water across capillary membranes was exclusively attributed to capillary and surrounding tissue hydrostatic pressures. Current physiologic understanding clarified that various types of permeable, fenestrated, and nonfenestrated capillaries exist throughout the body.

Third Spacing

As pressure and fluid volume increases, the limited expansion capacity of the abdominal cavity leads to compression of and reduced blood flow to the abdominal organs. Reductions in the vascular transmural pressure gradient and poor microvascular perfusion trigger activation and perpetuation of the inflammatory cascade. Subsequent release of inflammatory mediators promotes capillary leakage and extravascular fluid loss, or third spacing. The fluid inefficiently shifts out of the vascular space to collect in the collagen-mucopolysaccharide matrix in the interstitial space, lengthening the diffusion distance for oxygen and cellular metabolism nutrients, thus rendering it inaccessible for physiologic utilization.

Proper function of sodium-potassium pump, and its associated regulation of intracellular electrolytes, is also affected by fluid shifts, membrane disturbances, and pressure gradients. Leakage of sodium into the cells shifts water molecules into the cell, causing cellular swelling and spillage of intracellular contents. This damage further heightens the inflammatory cascade and increases edema. As plasma shifts and moves out of abdominal vascular circulation and into the peritoneal cavity, an increase in intraperitoneal hydrostatic pressure occurs. Early clinical detection of this fluid shift is rare.

Third spacing is further enhanced by multiple factors affecting the osmotic pressure gradient. Capillary hypertension facilitates the movement of low-protein fluid into the interstitial spaces and out of the tissues. Disruptions of the microvascular barrier (from trauma and the abdominal organ compression from rising pressure) lead further to an inefficient colloid osmotic pressure gradient. This also encourages the endothelial barrier to allow movement of protein-rich filtrate into tissue spaces. As the circulating levels of albumin declines, so does the colloid osmotic pressure gradient. Considering the deleterious effects of hypoproteinemia on edema etiology, careful consideration should be given when determining macromolecules in fluid infusions.

Clinical Considerations

Whether due to increased fluid volume, increased capillary hydrostatic pressure, decreased sodium levels, albumin losses, or increased capillary permeability, third-space edema is of particular concern in the peritoneal cavity due to expansive anatomic limitations and secondary systemic effects. Transcapillary flow barriers affect flow into the draining lymphatic vessels, leading to lymphatic system obstruction.[21] Third spacing occurs in 2 phases: the loss phase and the reabsorption phase.[20] The 24-hour to 72-hour loss phase is a critical concern in ACS patients, because proteins and fluids are moving out of the vascular space and into the interstitial space.

In patients who develop ACS, increased volume and increased capillary permeability are of primary concern to nurse clinicians. As discussed previously, this increase in permeability is often associated with release of proinflammatory cytokines and other inflammatory mediators, including histamines, bradykinin, and anaphylatoxins.[22] These molecules stimulate vasodilation while increasing capillary permeability, further promoting edema development. Typically, the endothelial barrier exerts restrictive properties on fluid movement, but increased microvascular permeability, rising interstitial fluid pressure, and vasodilation encourage continued fluid flux. Inflammatory states are also associated with infiltration of leukocytes into the tissues.

Ultimately, fluid volume excess and an increase in extracellular water are strongly correlated with the development of increased IAP.[23] In both third-spacing and capillary leak syndromes, an increase in extracellular water occurs. Thus, identifying patients at risk and ensuring early assessment of IAP are key to preventing the development of ACS and secondary organ system involvement.[17]

INTRA-ABDOMINAL HYPERTENSION AND ABDOMINAL COMPARTMENT SYNDROME TREATMENT CONSIDERATIONS

Current treatment of IAH and ACS is a multidisciplinary approach, including the astute assessment by and management skills of multiple health care clinicians. Critical care nurse clinicians are often front-line professionals and the first to notice an abnormal abdominal assessment. Advanced practice nurses, surgeons, dieticians, and therapists should be aware of the effects of ACS on the overall patient state of health. Early IAP management and efforts to relieve or decompress the abdomen are considered standard of care.[15] Each ACS case should be approached uniquely and interventions planned to achieve the best outcome for patients and to decrease overall mortality.

FLUID RESUSCITATION PRACTICE CHANGES

Nurse clinicians should note that recent, significant changes have been made to fluid resuscitation guidelines. Subsequently, it is hopeful that a reduction in the incidence of ACS occurs secondary to the implementation of these guidelines into resuscitative practice efforts. Recent guidelines have indicated the need to move away from excessive crystalloid fluid resuscitation due to the increase in pulmonary, cardiovascular, and abdominal mortality and morbidity.[24,25]

In a combat field study in the setting of hemorrhagic shock, instead of crystalloid fluids, clinicians should first consider whole blood, plasma products, packed red blood cells, or lactated Ringer solution for appropriate resuscitation.[25] Minimizing the use of normal saline with packed red blood cells infusions is also encouraged. Additionally, the use of Hextend (a plasma volume expander containing hetastarch) is recommended for shock states. Hextend (BioTime Inc, Alameda, CA, USA) should be supplemented with minimal crystalloid (lactated Ringer) infusion to maintain a target blood pressure above systolic 80 mm Hg to 90 mm Hg.[25]

More broadly, clinicians should consider DCR efforts with fluid resuscitation. This practice suggests replacing lost volume in an in-hospital setting with crystalloids, blood products, and platelets/plasma in a 1:1:1 ratio.[24] Overall, the consensus is that fluid resuscitative efforts should involve assessing the specific needs of a patient, including maintaining a palpable peripheral pulse, a minimum systolic blood pressure, and an appropriate level of consciousness.[24] Although definite efforts to move away from massive crystalloid infusions are apparent, the standard of care is still to infuse crystalloids but only to specific outcome parameters. Further research is needed in the form of controlled trials to determine the efficacy of using Hextend only, because current studies do not demonstrate improvement in mortality associated with this practice.[25]

In light of the new fluid resuscitation practice efforts, nurse clinicians should consider how these practice changes will affect a patient at risk for developing ACS. The WSACS guidelines address these new practices in several ways in the latest consensus document[15] (**Box 1**). A positive fluid balance has shown to increase complications and mortality specifically associated with ACS. It is recommended that a positive fluid balance be avoided in patients at risk for developing IAH/ACS. Secondly, diuretics are often used to maintain fluid balance in critically ill patients, and there is no evidence to support a change in this practice to improve outcomes for patients who may develop IAH or ACS. Third, albumin and Hextend are used to expand plasma volume and to improve oncotic pressure in critically ill patients. There is not enough evidence to support or

---

Box 1
World Society of the Abdominal Compartment Syndrome recommendations related to fluid resuscitation and balance in patients with or at risk of developing intra-abdominal hypertension or abdominal compartment syndrome

1. Avoid a positive fluid balance

2. No recommendation on the use of diuretics maintain fluid balance

3. No recommendation on the use of albumin as volume expander

4. Use DCR

refute this practice in relation to patients who develop IAH or ACS. DCR, as discussed previously, is the practice of judiciously using crystalloids and choosing more plasma/platelets/red blood cells in light of endpoint parameters, such as systolic blood pressure and presence of peripheral pulse. The recommendation is that DCR is beneficial to improve the risk and outcomes associated with IAH and ACS.

SUMMARY

In summary, ACS is a potentially deadly complication of increased abdominal pressure and fluid shifts. Nurse clinicians are aware that multiple approaches to fluid resuscitation exist for various patient needs. This article explores the basic pathophysiology of IAH/ACS related to fluid shifts, with specific guidelines for managing fluid resuscitation while considering the risk for developing IAH and ACS. Considering the significant and rapid mortality rates, every effort should be considered for evaluating the risk for development of IAH and ACS. The literature suggests considerable concern exists when excessive amounts of crystalloids are infused in an attempt to achieve fluid balance. Thus, recent evidence suggests that outcome-directed DCR efforts may achieve more appropriate patient outcomes and may reduce the likelihood that a patient develops IAH or ACS. Even though further rigorous study is needed to guide the definite practice of fluid resuscitation, nurse clinicians should consider this recent evidence to optimize care and outcomes.

Nurse professionals in all scopes of practice are uniquely advantageous for patients at high risk of developing IAH/ACS. A critical care bedside nurse most often notices initial changes in patient condition. A bedside nurse is responsible for obtaining and maintaining IAH and ACS monitoring. Advanced practice nurses, particularly when doctorally prepared, provide high-quality, evidence-based care and perhaps are best positioned to translate the latest evidence into care for these patients. In cases of these complex disease processes, APNs use acutely changing assessment data, then implement evidence-based care, as this article considers. Regardless of the nurse clinician's role; early identification and collaborative, multidisciplinary care are necessary to achieve appropriate fluid balance in critically ill patients at risk for or who develop IAH or ACS.

REFERENCES

1. Bailey J, Shapiro M. Abdominal compartment syndrome. Crit Care 2000;4:23–9.
2. Bradley SE, Bradley GP. The effect of increased abdominal pressure on renal function. J Clin Invest 1947;26:1010–5.
3. Emerson H. Intra-abdominal pressures. Arch Intern Med 1911;7:754–84.
4. Baggot MG. Abdominal blow-out; a concept. Curr Res Anesth Analg 1951;30:295–9.
5. Kron IL, Harman PK, Nolan SP. The measurement of intra-abdominal pressure as a criterion for abdominal re-exploration. Ann Surg 1984;199:28–30.
6. Sugrue M, Bauman A, Jones F, et al. Clinical examination is an inaccurate predictor of intraabdominal pressure. World J Surg 2002;26(12):1428.
7. Malbrain M. Different techniques to measure intra-abdominal pressure (IAP): time for a critical re-appraisal. Intensive Care Med 2004;30(3):357–71.
8. Malbrain ML. Abdominal pressure in the critically ill: measurement and clinical relevance. Intensive Care Med 1999;25(12):1453–8.
9. Kirkpatrick AW, Brenneman FD, McLean RF, et al. Is clinical examination an accurate indicator of raised intra-abdominal pressure in critically injured patients? Can J Surg 2000;43(3):207.

10. Gudmundsson F, Viste A, Gislason H, et al. Comparison of different methods for measuring intra-abdominal pressure. Intensive Care Med 2002;28(4):509–14.
11. De Potter T, Dits H, Malbrain M. Intra- and interobserver variability during in vitro validation of two novel methods for intra-abdominal pressure monitoring. Intensive Care Med 2005;31(5):747–51.
12. Cheatham ML, Safcsak K. Intraabdominal pressure: a revised method for measurement. J Am Coll Surg 1998;186(5):594–5.
13. Balogh Z, Jones F, D'Amours S, et al. Continuous intra-abdominal pressure measurement technique. Am J Surg 2004;188(6):679–84.
14. Cheatham M, White M, Sagraves S, et al. Abdominal perfusion pressure: a superior parameter in the assessment of intra-abdominal hypertension. J Trauma 2000;49(4):621–7.
15. Kirkpatrick A, Roberts D, De Waele J, et al. Intra-abdominal hypertension and the abdominal compartment syndrome: updated consensus definitions and clinical practice guidelines from the World Society of the abdominal compartment syndrome. Intensive Care Med 2013;39(7):1190–206.
16. Cheatham ML. Abdominal compartment syndrome: pathophysiology and definitions. Scand J Trauma Resusc Emerg Med 2009;17(1):10.
17. Harrell BR, Melander S. Identifying the association among risk factors and mortality in trauma patients with intra-abdominal hypertension and abdominal compartment syndrome. J Trauma Nurs 2012;19(3):182.
18. Harris H, Smith C. Understanding abdominal compartment syndrome. Nursing Critical Care 2013;8(3):45–7.
19. Imm A, Carlson RW. Fluid resuscitation in circulatory shock. Crit Care Clin 1993; 9(2):313–33.
20. Myburgh JA, Mythen MG. Resuscitation fluids. N Engl J Med 2013;369(13):1243.
21. Holcomb S. Third-spacing: when body fluid shifts. Nursing 2008;38(7):50–3.
22. Vigneau C, Haymann J, Khoury N, et al. An unusual evolution of the systemic capillary leak syndrome. Nephrol Dial Transplant 2002;17(3):492–4.
23. Dąbrowski W, Kotlinska-Hasiec E, Jaroszynski A, et al. Intra-abdominal pressure correlates with extracellular water content. PLoS One 2015;10(4):e0122193.
24. McSwain NE, Champion HR, Fabian TC, et al. State of the art of fluid resuscitation 2010: prehospital and immediate transition to the hospital. J Trauma 2011; 70(5 Suppl, 2010 Prehospital Fluid Resuscitation Supplement):S2–10.
25. Butler F, Holcomb J, Schreiber M, et al. Fluid resuscitation for hemorrhagic shock in tactical combat casualty care. J Spec Oper Med 2014;14(3):13–38.

Index

Note: Page numbers of article titles are in **boldface** type.

Nurs Clin N Am 52 (2017) 339–347
http://dx.doi.org/10.1016/S0029-6465(17)30048-8
0029-6465/17

nursing.theclinics.com

Moving?

Make sure your subscription moves with you!

To notify us of your new address, find your **Clinics Account Number** (located on your mailing label above your name), and contact customer service at:

Email: journalscustomerservice-usa@elsevier.com

800-654-2452 (subscribers in the U.S. & Canada)
314-447-8871 (subscribers outside of the U.S. & Canada)

Fax number: 314-447-8029

Elsevier Health Sciences Division
Subscription Customer Service
3251 Riverport Lane
Maryland Heights, MO 63043

*To ensure uninterrupted delivery of your subscription, please notify us at least 4 weeks in advance of move.

Printed and bound by CPI Group (UK) Ltd, Croydon, CR0 4YY

03/10/2024

01040390-0007